Human Systematic Anatomy
Learning Instructions and Problem Sets

主　编　Dong Weijiang　董炜疆

副主编　Jin Hui　靳　辉　Yang Pengbo　杨蓬勃

编　者（按姓氏笔画为序）

Feng Gaifeng　冯改丰　Lyu Haixia　吕海侠

Liu Jianxin　刘建新　Xu Jiehua　许杰华

Sun Tianze　孙天泽　Li Yueying　李月英

Yang Jie　杨　杰　Yang Weina　杨维娜

Yang Pengbo　杨蓬勃　Zhang Jianshui　张建水

Chen Guomin　陈国敏　Hu Ming　胡　明

Jia Ning　贾　宁　Qian Yihua　钱亦华

Dong Weijiang　董炜疆　Jin Hui　靳　辉

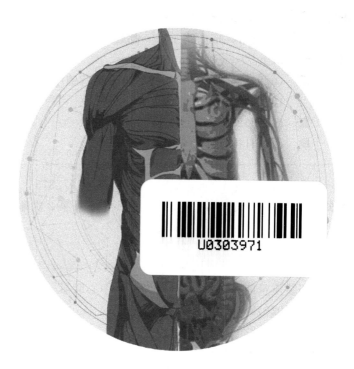

西安交通大学出版社
XI'AN JIAOTONG UNIVERSITY PRESS

国家一级出版社
全国百佳图书出版单位

图书在版编目(CIP)数据

人体系统解剖学学习指导与习题集＝Human Systematic Anatomy
Learning Instructions and Problem Sets：英文/董炜疆主编. —西安：
西安交通大学出版社,2019.8(2023.9 重印)
　ISBN 978 - 7 - 5693 - 1249 - 2

　Ⅰ.①人…　Ⅱ.①董…　Ⅲ.①系统解剖学-医学院校-教学参考
资料-英文　Ⅳ.①R322

中国版本图书馆 CIP 数据核字(2019)第 144234 号

书　　名	Human Systematic Anatomy Learning Instructions and Problem Sets
主　　编	董炜疆
责任编辑	杨　花　刘　攀

出版发行	西安交通大学出版社
	（西安市兴庆南路 1 号　邮政编码 710048）
网　　址	http://www.xjtupress.com
电　　话	（029）82668357　82667874（市场营销中心）
	（029）82668315（总编办）
传　　真	（029）82668280
印　　刷	西安日报社印务中心

开　　本	787mm×1092mm　1/16　　印张 17.875　　字数 445千字
版次印次	2019 年 8 月第 1 版　　2023 年 9 月第 2 次印刷
书　　号	ISBN 978 - 7 - 5693 - 1249 - 2
定　　价	52.00元

如发现印装质量问题,请与本社市场营销中心联系。
订购热线:(029)82665248　(029)82667874
投稿热线:(029)82668803
读者信箱:med_xjup@163.com

Preface

Human anatomy is the scientific study on the structure of human body, including its systems, organs and tissues. It is unquestionably crucial to any sciences regarding human health and medicine. As the first subject introduced to international students who study medicine in China, human anatomy not only lays the foundation for other basic medical subjects such as pathology and physiology, but also links to students' future clinical study and their future practice. For over 20 years, suffering from the lack of English versions of teaching and exercising materials, international students in our university have found it difficult to review human anatomy before the examination, let alone good scores. To enable international students to grapple the key knowledge of human anatomy in a relatively short time, teachers in department of human anatomy and histology & embryology elaborated on the plans and requirements, and compiled *Human Anatomy Problem Sets for International Students*. It supplements the general courses of human anatomy, providing guidance to international students, teachers and health workers alike.

This book is written according to the human anatomy teaching program and the newest version of *A Textbook of Human Anatomy*. It is arranged in the same pattern as the textbook, with content divided into chapters and sections. The number and difficulty of questions are varied according to the key points and teaching hours, covering the full content of textbook. Question types range from simple reciting to comprehension and application, including single choice, double choices, fill in the blanks, brief questions and in-detail questions, as well as interesting "problems in life". Model answers are attached to the end of each chapter, suitable as review reference and a tool to consolidate textbook knowledge.

Authors for this book are all devoted professors and teachers with years of experience in teaching of human anatomy. This book is for international students that major in all branches of medical science to study systematic anatomy.

Special thanks to School of International Education for their funding in the writing and publication of this book. Thanks to Xi'an Jiaotong University Press and Department of Human Anatomy & Histology and Embryology for their support and help.

We would also like to express thanks to the authors of the books we referred in the compilation of this book. Due to the limitations in our knowledge, omissions and errors can hardly be avoided. We welcome any criticisms and corrections from any users of this book, in order to improve it for the next edition.

CONTENTS

Part 1　The Locomotor System

Chapter 1　The Bones

Ⅰ. **Single choice（Choose the best answer among the following four choices, and write down the corresponding letter in bracket）**

1. Which of the following is the particular feature of the thoracic vertebrae? (　　)
   A. The spines are short and bifid.
   B. Each transverse process has the transverse foramen.
   C. The bodies are kidney-shaped in outline.
   D. Each side of vertebral bodies has a costal facet.

2. Which bone belongs to the long bone? (　　)
   A. Vertebra
   B. Sternum
   C. Femur
   D. Tarsal bone

3. Which bone does **not** belong to the flat bone? (　　)
   A. Rib
   B. Ulna
   C. Sternum
   D. Scapula

4. Which bone belongs to the short bone? (　　)
   A. Carpal bone
   B. Sacrum
   C. Tibia
   D. Parietal bone

5. Which bone belongs to the pneumatic bone? (　　)
   A. Temporal bone
   B. Maxilla
   C. Mandible
   D. Nasal bone

6. Which structure can produce blood cells? (　　)

   A. Bony substance
   B. Bone marrow
   C. Periosteum
   D. Nerve
7. Which structure performs the function of the regeneration of the bones? (   )
   A. Compact bone
   B. Spongy bone
   C. Periosteum
   D. Bone marrow
8. Which bone does **not** form the thoracic cage? (   )
   A. Rib
   B. Thoracic vertebra
   C. Sternum
   D. Sacrum
9. Which of the following is the feature of the atlas? (   )
   A. The spine is short and bifid.
   B. The transverse process has facets for articulation
   C. The body is small and kidney-shaped in outline.
   D. It has no body and no spine.
10. Which of the following is the particular feature of the lumbar vertebrae? (   )
    A. The body is small.
    B. Each transverse process has the transverse foramen.
    C. Each side of their bodies has a costal facet.
    D. The spines are thick and horizontal.
11. Which structure connects with the body of sternum? (   )
    A. Clavicle
    B. The first rib
    C. Thoracic vertebra
    D. The fifth rib
12. Which bone belongs to the cerebral cranium? (   )
    A. Maxilla
    B. Sphenoid bone
    C. Nasal bone
    D. Palatine bone
13. Which bone belongs to the facial cranium? (   )
    A. Nasal bone
    B. Parietal bone
    C. Temporal bone
    D. Occipital bone

14. Which bone forms the posteroinferior part of the bony nasal septum? (   )
    A. Nasal bone
    B. Ethmoid bone
    C. Vomer
    D. Inferior nasal concha
15. Which bone forms the upper and posterior part of the bony nasal septum? (   )
    A. Nasal bone
    B. Ethmoid bone
    C. Vomer
    D. Inferior nasal concha
16. Which bone does **not** form the anterior cranial fossa? (   )
    A. Frontal bone
    B. Sphenoid bone
    C. Temporal bone
    D. Ethmoid bone
17. Which bone forms the middle cranial fossa? (   )
    A. Occipital bone
    B. Parietal bone
    C. Temporal bone
    D. Frontal bone
18. Which bone forms both the middle and posterior cranial fossae? (   )
    A. Occipital bone
    B. Parietal bone
    C. Temporal bone
    D. Frontal bone
19. Which structure lies in the anterior cranial fossa? (   )
    A. Crista galli
    B. Foramen rotundum
    C. Jugular foramen
    D. Foramen magnum
20. The structure that lies in the middle cranial fossa is (   ).
    A. cribriform foramina
    B. hypophysial fossa
    C. jugular foramen
    D. inferior orbital fissure
21. Which of the following can be seen in the posterior cranial fossa? (   )
    A. Occipital condyle
    B. Internal acoustic pore
    C. Optic canal

    D. External occipital protuberance

22. Which of the following connects the middle cranial fossa with the orbit? (　　)
    A. superior orbital fissure
    B. inferior orbital fissure
    C. foramen rotundum
    D. foramen ovale

23. The anterior cranial fossa communicates with the nasal cavity by (　　).
    A. foramen rotundum
    B. foramen ovale
    C. cribriform foramina
    D. foramen magnum

24. The pathway connecting the posterior cranial fossa with the vertebral canal is
    (　　).
    A. foramen rotundum
    B. foramen ovale
    C. cribriform foramina
    D. foramen magnum

25. The pathway connecting the pterygopalatine fossa with the orbit is (　　).
    A. superior orbital fissure
    B. inferior orbital fissure
    C. cribriform foramina
    D. foramen magnum

26. The pathway connecting the infratemporal fossa with the orbit is (　　).
    A. superior orbital fissure
    B. inferior orbital fissure
    C. cribriform foramina
    D. foramen magnum

27. The following structures lie in the greater wing of sphenoid bone, **except** (　　).
    A. foramen rotundum
    B. foramen ovale
    C. foramen spinosum
    D. foramen magnum

28. Which bone does **not** possess the squamous part? (　　)
    A. Frontal bone
    B. Temporal bone
    C. Sphenoid bone
    D. Occipital bone

29. The coronal suture lies between (　　).
    A. frontal and parietal bones

    B. parietal and temporal bones

    C. parietal and occipital bones

    D. temporal and occipital bones

30. The sagittal suture lies between (   ).

    A. frontal and parietal bones

    B. parietal and temporal bones

    C. parietal and occipital bones

    D. two parietal bones

31. The lambdoid suture is formed by (   ).

    A. frontal and parietal bones

    B. parietal and temporal bones

    C. parietal and occipital bones

    D. temporal and occipital bones

32. The pterion is formed by the following bones, **except** (   ).

    A. frontal bone

    B. parietal bone

    C. temporal bone

    D. occipital bone

33. Which of the following does **not** belong to humerus? (   )

    A. Trochlear notch

    B. Deltoid tuberosity

    C. Trochlea

    D. Groove for ulnar nerve

34. Which one belongs to the false rib? (   )

    A. The first rib

    B. The third rib

    C. The eighth rib

    D. The second rib

35. About the scapula, which of the statements is **not** true? (   )

    A. It is a flat bone.

    B. It has three borders, three angles and three surfaces.

    C. The anterior surface is concave and known as subscapular fossa.

    D. The inferior angle is opposite to the seventh rib or the seventh intercostal space.

36. Which of the following does **not** lie in the proximal end of the ulna? (   )

    A. Trochlear notch

    B. Olecranon

    C. Coronoid process

    D. Styloid process

37. Which bone belongs to the distal row of carpal bones? (   )

    A. Scaphoid bone

    B. Lunate bone

    C. Hamate bone

    D. Pisiform bone

38. About the radius, which of the statements is **not** true? (   )

    A. It is a long bone.

    B. The proximal end includes a head, neck and tuberosity.

    C. The lateral margin of the shaft is interosseous border.

    D. The distal end has a thick styloid process.

39. Which structure does **not** belong to the ilium? (   )

    A. Iliac crest

    B. Obturator foramen

    C. Arcuate line

    D. Anterior superior iliac spine

40. The acetabulum is fused by the body of (   ).

    A. ilium and pubis

    B. pubis and ischium

    C. ilium and ischium

    D. ilium, pubis and ischium

41. The obturator foramen is enclosed by (   ).

    A. ilium and pubis

    B. pubis and ischium

    C. ilium and ischium

    D. ilium, pubis and ischium

42. About the femur, which of the following is **not** true? (   )

    A. It is the longest bone in the body.

    B. It has two necks, namely anatomical neck and surgical neck.

    C. Between the neck and body, there are two trochanters.

    D. The lower end can articulate with tibia and patella.

43. Which structure does **not** belong to the tibia? (   )

    A. Medial condyle

    B. Intercondylar fossa

    C. Medial malleolus

    D. Fibular notch

44. About the fibula, which statement is **not** true? (   )

    A. It is a long bone.

    B. It is located on the lateral side of the tibia.

    C. The lower end forms lateral malleolus.

    D. It can articulate with the femur, tibia and talus.

45. About the orbit, which of the statements is **not** true? (   )

    A. It is shaped like a four-sided pyramid.

    B. It has an apex, a base and four walls.

    C. It communicates with the anterior cranial fossa through the optic canal.

    D. It communicates with the nasal cavity through the nasolacrimal canal.

46. Which bone does **not** form the orbit? (   )

    A. Temporal bone

    B. Frontal bone

    C. Sphenoid bone

    D. Maxilla

47. Which wall of the orbit does the lacrimal gland lie in? (   )

    A. Superior wall

    B. Inferior wall

    C. Medial wall

    D. Lateral wall

48. Which bone forms the roof of the bony nasal cavity? (   )

    A. Nasal bone

    B. Frontal bone

    C. Ethmoid bone

    D. Maxilla

49. Which of the paranasal sinus opens into the superior nasal meatus? (   )

    A. Maxillary sinus

    B. Frontal sinus

    C. Sphenoidal sinus

    D. Ethmoidal sinus (posterior group)

50. About the bony nasal cavity, which of the statements is **not** true? (   )

    A. It is divided into two spaces by bony nasal septum.

    B. It has two anterior nasal apertures and one posterior nasal aperture.

    C. It communicates with the anterior cranial fossa by cribriform foramina.

    D. Superior, middle and inferior nasal conchae lie on the lateral wall of the cavity.

51. Where does the sphenoidal sinus open into? (   )

    A. Superior nasal meatus

    B. Middle nasal meatus

    C. Inferior nasal meatus

    D. Sphenoethmoidal recess

52. Where does the frontal sinus open into? (   )

    A. Superior nasal meatus

    B. Middle nasal meatus

    C. Inferior nasal meatus

D. Sphenoethmoidal recess

53. Which structure does **not** belong to the maxilla? (   )

A. Maxillary sinus

B. Frontal process

C. Zygomatic process

D. Coronoid process

54. Which structure does **not** belong to the mandible? (   )

A. Mental foramen

B. Alveolar arch

C. Coronoid process

D. Zygomatic process

55. Which part of temporal bone forms the middle and posterior cranial fossae? (   )

A. Squamous part

B. Mastoid part

C. Tympanic part

D. Petrous part

56. Which part of sphenoid bone can **not** be seen in the internal aspect of the skull? (   )

A. Body

B. Greater wing

C. Lesser wing

D. Pterygoid lamina

Ⅱ. Double choices (Choose the two best answers among the following choices, and write down the corresponding letters in bracket)

1. Which bones belong to the flat bone? (   )

A. Rib

B. Ulna

C. Vertebra

D. Sternum

E. Sphenoid bone

2. Which structures belong to the thoracic vertebra? (   )

A. Transverse foramen

B. Costal fovea

C. Dens

D. Auricular surface

E. Transverse costal fovea

3. Which bones belong to the irregular bone? (   )

A. Rib

   B. Ulna

   C. Vertebra

   D. Sternum

   E. Sphenoid bone

4. Paranasal sinuses lie in the (　　).

   A. palatine bone

   B. temporal bone

   C. maxilla

   D. mandible

   E. frontal bone

5. About the cervical vertebrae, which ones of the following statements are **not** true?
(　　)

   A. The body is small.

   B. The vertebral foramen is relatively large.

   C. All of the spines are short and bifid.

   D. Each transverse process has the transverse foramen.

   E. Each side of their bodies has a costal facet.

6. Which bones belong to the shoulder girdle? (　　)

   A. Humerus

   B. Ulna

   C. Scapula

   D. Sternum

   E. Clavicle

7. Which structures do **not** belong to the scapula? (　　)

   A. Glenoid cavity

   B. Deltoid tuberosity

   C. Coracoid process

   D. Olecranon

   E. Acromion

8. Which bones do **not** form the bony pelvis? (　　)

   A. Lumbar vertebra

   B. Sacrum

   C. Coccyx

   D. Hip bone

   E. Femur

9. Which ones of the following do **not** lie in the proximal end of the femur? (　　)

   A. Medial condyle

   B. Popliteal surface

   C. Femoral head

D. Greater trochanter

E. Lesser trochanter

10. The bones of the skull are closely fitted together by sutures or cartilages, **except** ( ).

A. frontal bone

B. hyoid bone

C. maxilla

D. mandible

E. palatine bone

11. The paired cerebral bones are ( ).

A. frontal bone

B. parietal bone

C. temporal bone

D. occipital bone

E. ethmoid bone

12. The unpaired facial bones are ( ).

A. nasal bone

B. mandible

C. lacrimal bone

D. hyoid bone

E. palatine bone

13. The hard palate is formed by ( ).

A. maxilla

B. mandible

C. lacrimal bone

D. hyoid bone

E. palatine bone

14. The bony nasal septum is formed by ( ).

A. nasal bone

B. ethmoid bone

C. vomer

D. inferior nasal concha

E. palatine bone

15. The anterior cranial fossa is formed by orbital plate of frontal bone and ( ).

A. greater wings of sphenoid bone

B. lesser wings of sphenoid bone

C. cribriform plate of ethmoid bone

D. perpendicular plate of ethmoid bone

E. ethmoidal labyrinth

16. The middle cranial fossa is formed by (   ).

   A. occipital bone

   B. parietal bone

   C. temporal bone

   D. frontal bone

   E. sphenoid bone

17. The pathways connecting the middle cranial fossa with the orbit are (   ).

   A. superior orbital fissure

   B. inferior orbital fissure

   C. foramen rotundum

   D. foramen ovale

   E. optic canal

18. The inferior orbital fissure connects the orbit with (   ).

   A. anterior cranial fossa

   B. middle cranial fossa

   C. posterior cranial fossa

   D. pterygopalatine fossa

   E. infratemporal fossa

19. The structures lying on the external aspect of the base of skull are (   ).

   A. crista galli

   B. hypophysial fossa

   C. jugular foramen

   D. superior orbital fissure

   E. occipital condyle

20. The following structures belong to the posterior cranial fossa, **except** (   ).

   A. internal acoustic pore

   B. foramen rotundum

   C. jugular foramen

   D. foramen magnum

   E. external acoustic pore

Ⅲ. Fill the blanks (Fill the most appropriate words in the blanks)

1. The axial bone contains _____ and _____.

2. According to the shape, bones are classified into _____, _____, _____ and _____.

3. Bony substance includes _____ and _____.

4. The two layers of periosteum are _____ and _____.

5. Bone marrow contains _____ and _____.

6. The bones of trunk include _____, _____ and _____.

7. The costal arch is formed by the _____ , _____ and _____ ribs.

8. The sternum consists of _____ , _____ and _____ three parts.

9. The shoulder girdle contains _____ and _____ .

10. The bones of hand include three parts, _____ , _____ and _____ .

11. The hip bone of a newborn consists of three components, _____ , _____ and _____ .

12. Between two trochanters of the femur, on the anterior surface is _____ , on the posterior surface is _____ .

13. Vertebra is formed by _____ anteriorly and _____ posteriorly, the foramen between these two parts is _____ .

14. The unpaired cerebral bones are _____ , _____ , _____ and _____ .

15. Zygomatic arch is formed by _____ and _____ .

16. The foramina on the greater wing of sphenoid bone are _____ , _____ and _____ .

17. Two processes on the superior end of ramus of mandible are _____ and _____ .

18. The sphenoid bone is formed by _____ , _____ , _____ and _____ four parts.

19. The palatine bone consists of _____ and _____ two parts, and _____ forms the posterior part of the bony palate.

20. Four processes of maxilla are _____ , _____ , _____ and _____ .

IV. Answer questions briefly

1. Please describe the shape and classification of bones.
2. Please describe the structure of bones.
3. Please describe the general features of the vertebrae.
4. Please describe the main characteristics of cervical vertebra.
5. Please describe the main characteristics of thoracic vertebra.
6. Please describe the main characteristics of lumbar vertebra.
7. Please describe the features of the scapula.
8. Please describe the features of the mandible.
9. Please describe the features of the femur.
10. Please describe the groups and names of bones of skull.

V. Answer questions in detail

1. Please describe the shape, structures and communications of the orbit.
2. Please describe the formation, main structures and communications of the middle cranial fossa.
3. Please describe the location and openings of the paranasal sinuses.

4. Please describe the structures of the bony nasal cavity.

5. Please describe the features of the hip bone.

VI. **Problems in life**

1. When astronauts are subjected to prolonged weightlessness in space, why do their bones begin to degenerate and lose calcium and other minerals?

2. What are "shin splint"?

Chapter 2　The Joints

I. **Single choice（Choose the best answer among the following four choices, and write down the corresponding letter in bracket）**

1. Which of the following does **not** belong to the synarthrosis? (　　)
   A. Suture
   B. Syndesmosis
   C. Symphysis
   D. Synovial joint

2. Which of the following belongs to the fibrous joint? (　　)
   A. Synchondrosis
   B. Syndesmosis
   C. Symphyses
   D. Synovial joint

3. Which of the following belongs to the cartilaginous joint? (　　)
   A. Synchondrosis
   B. Syndesmosis
   C. Suture
   D. Synosteosis

4. Which of the bone's connections is a synosteosis? (　　)
   A. Humerus and ulna
   B. Ulna and radius
   C. Two pubic bones
   D. Ilium, pubis and ischium

5. The following structures belong to the essential structures of a synovial joint, **except** (　　).
   A. articular surface
   B. articular disc
   C. articular capsule
   D. articular cavity

6. Which of the following does **not** belong to the accessory structure of a synovial joint? (　　)
   A. Articular disc
   B. Articular cavity
   C. Synovial fold
   D. Articular labrum

7. About the flexion and extension, which of the statement is correct? (　　)

    A. These movements are performed in the coronal axis.

    B. These movements are performed in the sagittal axis.

    C. These movements are performed in the vertical axis.

    D. The movement between neighboring arches of vertebrae is of this type.

8. About the joint movements, which of the statement is correct? (　　)

    A. The movement between carpal bones is rotation.

    B. Flexion and extension can be occurred in shoulder joint.

    C. The movement between ulna and radius is gliding movement.

    D. The adduction and abduction are performed in the coronary axis.

9. Which movement can be performed in the sagittal axis? (　　)

    A. Rotation

    B. Flexion and extension

    C. Adduction and abduction

    D. Gliding movement

10. Which movement can be performed in the coronary axis? (　　)

    A. Rotation

    B. Flexion and extension

    C. Adduction and abduction

    D. Gliding movement

11. Which movement can be performed in the vertical axis? (　　)

    A. Rotation

    B. Flexion and extension

    C. Adduction and abduction

    D. Gliding movement

12. Shoulder joint can do all of the following movements, **except** (　　).

    A. rotation

    B. flexion and extension

    C. adduction and abduction

    D. gliding movement

13. About the uniaxial joints, which of the statements is correct? (　　)

    A. It is formed by one bone.

    B. Movement is around only one axis.

    C. It has three types, hinge joint, pivot joint and saddle joint.

    D. The humeroulnar joint belongs to the pivot joint.

14. About the biaxial joints, which of the statements is **wrong**? (　　)

    A. Movement is around two axes.

    B. Two axes lie at approximately 90° to one another.

    C. It has two types, ellipsoid joint and saddle joint.

    D. The carpometacarpal joint of thumb belongs to the ellipsoid joint.

15. About the polyaxial joints, which of the statements is **wrong**? (　　)

    A. Movement is around innumerable axes.

    B. It has three types, ball and socket joint, plane joint and saddle joint.

    C. Ball and socket joint is the freest moving synovial joint.

    D. Plane joint permits only little of movement.

16. Which of the following belongs to the uniaxial joint? (　　)

    A. Hinge joint

    B. Ellipsoidal joint

    C. Ball and socket joint

    D. Plane joint

17. Which of the following belongs to the biaxial joint? (　　)

    A. Hinge joint

    B. Ellipsoid joint

    C. Ball and socket joint

    D. Plane joint

18. Which of the following belongs to the polyaxial joint? (　　)

    A. Hinge joint

    B. Ellipsoid joint

    C. Ball and socket joint

    D. Pivot joint

19. Which of the following belongs to the ball and socket joint? (　　)

    A. Shoulder joint

    B. Knee joint

    C. Humeroulnar joint

    D. Wrist joint

20. Which of the following belongs to the hinge joint? (　　)

    A. Hip joint

    B. Shoulder joint

    C. Humeroulnar joint

    D. Wrist joint

21. Which of the following belongs to the pivot joint? (　　)

    A. Knee joint

    B. Radioulnar joint

    C. Humeroulnar joint

    D. Wrist joint

22. Which of the following belongs to the ellipsoid joint? (　　)

    A. Knee joint

    B. Radioulnar joint

C. Humeroulnar joint

D. Wrist joint

23. Which of the following does **not** belong to the articulations of the vertebral column?
(　　)

A. Ligament

B. Suture

C. Intervertebral disc

D. Synovial joint

24. The joints of the vertebral bodies contain the following types, **except** (　　).

A. intervertebral disc

B. anterior longitudinal ligament

C. posterior longitudinal ligament

D. zygapophysial joint

25. Which of the following does **not** belong to the joints of the vertebral arches? (　　)

A. Anterior longitudinal ligament

B. Interspinal ligament

C. Supraspinal ligament

D. Zygapophysial joint

26. The ligament which connects the adjacent vertebral laminae is (　　).

A. interspinal ligament

B. intertransverse ligament

C. yellow ligament

D. supraspinal ligament

27. The long ligament belongs to the joints of the vertebral arches is (　　).

A. anterior longitudinal ligament

B. interspinal ligament

C. supraspinal ligament

D. yellow ligament

28. The ligament which connects the adjacent transverse processes is (　　).

A. interspinal ligament

B. intertransverse ligament

C. yellow ligament

D. supraspinal ligament

29. About the intervertebral disc, which of the statements is **wrong**? (　　)

A. It is a symphysis between vertebral bodies.

B. It consists of an outer annulus fibrosus and an inner nucleus pulposus.

C. Annulus fibrosus is tough and nucleus pulposus is pliable.

D. Prolapsed disc means the annulus fibrosus protruding into the vertebral canal.

30. About the shoulder joint, which of the statement is **wrong**? (　　)

A. It is a ball and socket joint.

B. It links the head of humerus to the glenoid cavity of the scapula.

C. The glenoid labrum lies within the articular cavity.

D. The dislocation of the humeral head usually occurs in the superior direction.

31. Which of the following is **not** enclosed in the articular capsule of shoulder joint?
(   )

A. Head of humerus

B. Glenoid cavity of the scapula

C. Glenoid labrum

D. Tendon of the short head of the biceps

32. The following structures form the coracoacromial arch, **except** (   ).

A. coracoid process

B. coracoacromial ligament

C. spine of scapula

D. acromion

33. The following structures can reinforce the shoulder joint, **except** (   ).

A. coracohumeral ligament

B. coracoacromial ligament

C. tendinous cuff

D. ulnar collateral ligament

34. About the elbow joint, which of the statements is **wrong**? (   )

A. It is a compound synovial joint.

B. It is formed by three joints.

C. The articular capsule is thin and loose anteriorly and posteriorly.

D. As a whole, the elbow joint is a biaxial joint.

35. Which of the following belongs to the ball and socket joint? (   )

A. Humeroulnar joint

B. Humeroradial joint

C. Proximal radioulnar joint

D. Elbow joint as a whole

36. Which of the following belongs to the hinge joint? (   )

A. Humeroulnar joint

B. Humeroradial joint

C. Proximal radioulnar joint

D. Elbow joint as a whole

37. Which of the following belongs to the pivot joint? (   )

A. Humeroulnar joint

B. Humeroradial joint

C. Proximal radioulnar joint

D. Elbow joint as a whole

38. Which of the following is **not** enclosed in the articular capsule of elbow joint?
    (　　)
    A. Trochlea of the humerus and trochlear notch of ulna
    B. Capitulum of humerus and the upper concave surface of the radial head
    C. Head of the ulna and the ulnar notch of the radius
    D. Head of the radius and the radius notch of the ulna

39. Which of the following can hold the head of radius? (　　)
    A. Articular capsule of elbow joint
    B. Ulnar collateral ligament
    C. Radial collateral ligament
    D. Annular ligament

40. Which of the following contains the articular disc? (　　)
    A. Shoulder joint
    B. Ankle joint
    C. Sternoclavicular joint
    D. Elbow joint

41. Which of the following contains the articular labrum? (　　)
    A. Shoulder joint
    B. Ankle joint
    C. Sternoclavicular joint
    D. Elbow joint

42. Which of the following contains the articular meniscus? (　　)
    A. Shoulder joint
    B. Knee joint
    C. Sternoclavicular joint
    D. Elbow joint

43. Which of the ligaments belongs to the intracapsular ligament? (　　)
    A. Ulnar collateral ligament
    B. Tibial collateral ligament
    C. Patellar ligament
    D. Anterior cruciate ligament

44. Which of the ligaments belongs to the extracapsular ligament? (　　)
    A. Anterior cruciate ligament
    B. Posterior cruciate ligament
    C. Patellar ligament
    D. Ligament of head of femur

45. About the hip joint, which of the statement is **wrong**? (　　)
    A. It is a ball and socket joint.

      B. It links the femoral head to the fossa of the acetabulum.

      C. The acetabular labrum lies within the articular cavity.

      D. It is easier to dislocate than the shoulder joint.

46. Which of the following is **not** enclosed in the articular capsule of hip joint? (　　)

      A. Femoral head

      B. Fossa of acetabulum

      C. Transverse acetabular ligament

      D. Intertrochanteric crest

47. Which of the ligaments lies surround the femoral neck? (　　)

      A. Transverse acetabular ligament

      B. Ligament of head of femur

      C. Zona orbicularis

      D. Iliofemoral ligament

48. Which of the ligaments does **not** belong to the knee joint? (　　)

      A. Anterior cruciate ligament

      B. Tibial collateral ligament

      C. Patellar ligament

      D. Iliofemoral ligament

49. About the knee joint, which one is **incorrect**? (　　)

      A. It is the largest and most complicated joint in the body.

      B. It is formed by the joints among femur, tibia, fibula and patella.

      C. The anterior cruciate ligament arises in front of the intercondylar eminence of the tibia.

      D. The medial meniscus is larger and less curved than the lateral meniscus.

50. Which of the following is **not** enclosed in the articular capsule of knee joint? (　　)

      A. Head of fibula

      B. Patella

      C. Cruciate ligament

      D. Medial meniscus

51. Which of the accessory structures of the synovial joint does **not** belong to the knee joint? (　　)

      A. Ligament

      B. Articular labrum

      C. Meniscus

      D. Synovial bursa

52. Which of the following joints contains the intracapsular ligament? (　　)

      A. Shoulder joint

      B. Ankle joint

      C. Sternoclavicular joint

D. Hip joint

53. Which of the following does **not** form the lesser sciatic foramen? (   )

    A. Greater sciatic notch

    B. Lesser sciatic notch

    C. Sacrotuberous ligament

    D. Sacrospinous ligament

54. About the pelvis, which of the statement is **wrong**? (   )

    A. Bony pelvis is formed by the sacrum, coccyx and two hip bones.

    B. It is divided into a greater pelvis and a lesser pelvis by the terminal line.

    C. The greater pelvis is the true pelvis and has two apertures.

    D. The superior aperture of the lesser pelvis is the terminal line.

55. About the sexual differences of pelvis, which of the statements is **wrong**? (   )

    A. Female pelvic cavity is wider and shorter than in a male.

    B. The pelvic inlet is heart-shaped in the male, oval in the female.

    C. The subpubic angle is narrow in male, wide in female.

    D. The inferior pelvic aperture is relatively large in male.

56. About the ankle joint, which of the statements is **wrong**? (   )

    A. It is a hinge joint.

    B. It links the tibia and fibula to the trochlea of the talus.

    C. The movement of the ankle joint are dorsiflexion and plantar flexion.

    D. The joint is more stable in the plantar flexed position.

57. Which bone does **not** form the articular surface of the wrist joint? (   )

    A. Scaphoid bone

    B. Lunate bone

    C. Triangular bone

    D. Pisiform bone

58. About the wrist joint, which of the statements is **wrong**? (   )

    A. It is a biaxial joint.

    B. It is a typical ellipsoid joint.

    C. The capsule is loose.

    D. The movements are flexion, extension, rotation and circumduction.

59. The mandible is connected with the cranial bones by (   ).

    A. suture

    B. synchondrosis

    C. synostosis

    D. synovial joint

60. About the temporomandibular joint, which of the statements is **wrong**? (   )

    A. It is a complex joint.

    B. The articular tubercle of temporal bone is enclosed in the articular capsule.

    C. The articular cavity has an articular disc.

    D. The mandible can be dislocated forwards and backwards.

II. Double choices (Choose the two best answers among the following choices, and write down the corresponding letters in bracket)

1. Which ones of the following belong to the fibrous joint? (   )

    A. Suture

    B. Intervertebral disc

    C. Interosseous membrane

    D. Acetabulum

    E. Shoulder joint

2. Which ones of the following belong to the cartilaginous joint? (   )

    A. Coronal suture

    B. Intervertebral disc

    C. Acetabulum

    D. Pubic symphysis

    E. Patellar ligament

3. The connections between ulna and radius include (   ).

    A. suture

    B. synostosis

    C. syndesmosis

    D. symphysis

    E. synovial joint

4. Which ones of the following belong to the accessory structures of a synovial joint? (   )

    A. Articular disc

    B. Articular cavity

    C. Synovial fold

    D. Articular capsule

    E. Articular surface

5. Which ones of the following belong to the essential structures of a synovial joint? (   )

    A. Articular disc

    B. Articular cavity

    C. Synovial fold

    D. Articular labrum

    E. Articular surface

6. About the articular capsule, which ones of the statements are correct? (   )

    A. It has two layers, synovial membrane and fibrous membrane.

B. The outer layer is synovial membrane.

C. Fibrous membrane is dense and riched in blood vessels and nerves.

D. Synovial membrane invests the surface of articular cartilages.

E. Articular cavity lies between synovial and fibrous membranes.

7. About the articular cavity, which ones of the statements are correct? (   )

　A. It is a closed cavity.

　B. It is formed by synovial membrane and fibrous membrane.

　C. It is formed by synovial membrane and articular cartilage.

　D. It contains a lot of synovia.

　E. Its pressure is equal to the atmospheric pressure.

8. Which movements can be performed in the sagittal axis? (   )

　A. Rotation

　B. Adduction

　C. Abduction

　D. Flexion

　E. Extension

9. Which ones of the following belong to the uniaxial joint? (   )

　A. Hinge joint

　B. Ellipsoidal joint

　C. Ball and socket joint

　D. Plane joint

　E. Pivot joint

10. Which ones of the following belong to the biaxial joint? (   )

　A. Hinge joint

　B. Ellipsoid joint

　C. Ball and socket joint

　D. Plane joint

　E. Saddle joint

11. Which ones of the following belong to the polyaxial joint? (   )

　A. Hinge joint

　B. Ellipsoid joint

　C. Ball and socket joint

　D. Pivot joint

　E. Plane joint

12. The ligaments associated with the vertebral body are (   ).

　A. interspinal ligament

　B. intertransverse ligament

　C. yellow ligament

　D. anterior longitudinal ligament

     E. posterior longitudinal ligament

13. The short ligaments belong to the joints of the vertebral arches are (   ).

     A. anterior longitudinal ligament

     B. interspinal ligament

     C. supraspinal ligament

     D. yellow ligament

     E. posterior longitudinal ligament

14. Which ones of the following contain the articular disc? (   )

     A. Shoulder joint

     B. Ankle joint

     C. Sternoclavicular joint

     D. Elbow joint

     E. Wrist joint

15. Which ones of the following contain the articular labrum? (   )

     A. Shoulder joint

     B. Ankle joint

     C. Sternoclavicular joint

     D. Elbow joint

     E. Hip joint

16. Which ones of the following contain the intracapsular ligament? (   )

     A. Hip joint

     B. Knee joint

     C. Wrist joint

     D. Shoulder joint

     E. Sternoclavicular joint

17. Shoulder joint is formed by (   ).

     A. head of humerus

     B. trochlea of humerus

     C. capitulum of humerus

     D. glenoid cavity of scapula

     E. articular facet of acromion

18. The proximal radioulnar joint is formed by (   ).

     A. trochlear notch of ulna

     B. head of radius

     C. radius notch of the ulna

     D. head of ulna

     E. ulnar notch of the radius

19. Which ones of the following form the greater sciatic foramen? (   )

     A. Greater sciatic notch

B. Lesser sciatic notch

C. Sacrotuberous ligament

D. Sacrospinous ligament

E. Pubic arch

20. Which structures do **not** form the articular surfaces of the knee joint? (   )

A. Head of femur

B. Medial and lateral condyles of femur

C. Patella

D. Head of fibula

E. Medial and lateral condyles of tibia

Ⅲ. **Fill the blanks** (**Fill the most appropriate words in the blanks**)

1. The synarthrosis consists of _____, _____ and _____.

2. Three types of fibrous joints are _____, _____ and _____.

3. The cartilaginous joint consists of _____ and _____.

4. The essential structures of a synovial joint include _____, _____, and _____.

5. The accessory structures of a synovial join include _____, _____, _____ and _____.

6. The uniaxial joint consists of _____ and _____.

7. The biaxial joint consists of _____ and _____.

8. The polyaxial joint consists of _____ and _____.

9. The costotransverse joint unites the _____ with the _____.

10. The thoracic cage is formed by _____, _____, _____ and the connections between them.

11. The intervertebral disc is composed of peripheral _____ and central _____.

12. The shoulder joint is formed by linking the _____ to _____.

13. Four physiological curvatures of vertebral column are _____, _____, _____ and _____.

14. Elbow joint contains _____, _____ and _____ three joints.

15. The inferior pelvic aperture is bounded behind by the _____, laterally by the _____ and _____, and anteriorly by the _____ and _____.

16. The lesser sciatic foramen is formed by _____, _____ and _____.

17. The hip joint is formed by linking the _____ to _____.

18. The intracapsular ligaments of knee joint are _____ and _____.

19. The joints which have the articular labrum are _____ and _____.

20. The joints which have the intracapsular ligaments are _____ and _____.

IV. Answer questions briefly

1. Please describe the definition and classification of the joint.
2. Please describe the essential structures of a synovial joint.
3. Please describe the accessory structures of a synovial joint.
4. Please describe the joints of the vertebral bodies.
5. Please describe the joints of the vertebral arches.
6. Please describe the composition and movements of the shoulder joint.
7. Please describe the composition and movements of the elbow joint.
8. Please describe the composition and movements of the hip joint.
9. Please describe the composition and movements of the knee joint.
10. Please describe the vertebral column as a whole.

V. Answer questions in detail

1. Please describe the essential and accessory structures of a synovial joint.
2. Please describe the articulations of the lumbar vertebrae.
3. Please describe the composition, characteristics and movements of the shoulder joint.
4. Please describe the composition, characteristics and movements of the hip joint.
5. Please describe the composition, characteristics and movements of the knee joint.

VI. Problems in life

What causes the "popping" sound when you crack your knuckles?

Chapter 3　The Muscles

Ⅰ. **Single choice (Choose the best answer among the following four choices, and write down the corresponding letter in bracket)**

1. The morphology of skeletal muscles does **not** include (　　).
   A. long muscle
   B. short muscle
   C. pennate muscle
   D. orbicular muscle

2. About the fascia, which of the statements is **wrong**? (　　)
   A. It is one of the supplementary structures of skeletal muscles.
   B. It contains superficial and deep fasciae.
   C. Superficial fascia lies beneath the cutis.
   D. Deep fascia is loose and contains fat, blood vessels and nerves.

3. Which of the following is **not** the supplementary structures of skeletal muscles?
   (　　)
   A. Tendon
   B. Fascia
   C. Synovial bursa
   D. Sesamoid bone

4. About the deep fascia, which of the statements is **wrong**? (　　)
   A. It is a dense, inelastic fibrous membrane.
   B. It lies beneath the superficial fascia.
   C. It forms intermuscular septa to separate the groups of muscles.
   D. At arm and forearm, it forms retinaculum to maintain the underlying tendons.

5. Which of the following does **not** belong to the masticatory muscles? (　　)
   A. Buccinator
   B. Temporalis
   C. Masseter
   D. Medial pterygoid

6. About the occipitofrontalis, which of the statements is **wrong**? (　　)
   A. It is a facial muscle.
   B. It covers almost whole of calvaria.
   C. It has two bellies and one epicranial aponeurosis.
   D. Epicranial aponeurosis is closely connected with the cutis and pericranium.

7. About the insertion of masticatory muscles, which of the statements is **wrong**?

(   )

A. Masseter is inserted to the head of mandible.

B. Temporalis is inserted to the coronoid process of mandible.

C. Medial pterygoid is inserted to the medial surface near the angle of mandible.

D. Lateral pterygoid is inserted to the neck of mandible.

8. Which of the muscles can open the mouth? (   )

A. Masseter

B. Temporalis

C. Medial pterygoid

D. Lateral pterygoid

9. Which of the following does **not** belong to the suprahyoid muscles? (   )

A. Digastric

B. Omohyoid

C. Mylohyoid

D. Geniohyoid

10. Which of the following belongs to the infrahyoid muscles? (   )

A. Platysma

B. Temporalis

C. Sternohyoid

D. Mylohyoid

11. About the sternocleidomastoid, which of the statements is **wrong**? (   )

A. It is one of the superficial muscles of the neck.

B. It arises from the manubrium and medial one-third of the clavicle.

C. It is inserted into the styloid process of the temporal bone.

D. Acting alone, the face is rotated to the opposite side.

12. The scalene fissure lies between (   ).

A. scalenus anterior and scalenus medius

B. scalenus anterior and scalenus posterior

C. scalenus medius and scalenus posterior

D. scalenus posterior and levator scapula

13. Which of the following is **not** the origin of the trapezius? (   )

A. External occipital protuberance

B. Spine of cervical vertebrae

C. Spine of thoracic vertebrae

D. Spine of lumbar vertebrae

14. Which of the movements of the shoulder joint can **not** be done by latissimus dorsi? (   )

A. Extension

B. Adduction

C. Abduction

D. Medial rotation

15. Trapezius can do the following movements, **except** (   ).

A. raising the scapula.

B. descending the scapula.

C. retracting and rotating the scapula.

D. flexing the head.

16. Which of the following does **not** belong to the extrinsic thoracic muscles? (   )

A. Pectoralis major

B. Pectoralis minor

C. Deltoid

D. Serratus anterior

17. The principal muscle of inspiration is (   ).

A. pectoralis major

B. pectoralis minor

C. diaphragm

D. intercostales interni

18. About the pectoralis major, which of the statement is **wrong**? (   )

A. It arises from the medial half of clavicle, sternum and upper six costal cartilages.

B. It is inserted into the crest of greater tubercle of humerus.

C. It can adduct, flex and medial rotate the arm.

D. When the arms are fixed, it draws the body downward.

19. About the intercostal muscles, which of the statements is right? (   )

A. Intercostales externi elevate the ribs and help to inspirate.

B. Intercostales externi elevate the ribs and help to expirate.

C. Intercostales interni elevate the ribs and help to inspirate.

D. Intercostales interni elevate the ribs and help to expirate.

20. Which of the following can drop the ribs? (   )

A. Serratus anterior

B. Intercostales externi

C. Diaphragm

D. Intercostales interni

21. About the diaphragm, which of the statements is **wrong**? (   )

A. It lies between the thoracic and abdominal cavities.

B. It consists of muscular fibers and central tendon.

C. The muscular fibers are divided into sternal and costal parts.

D. It is the principal muscle of inspiration.

22. The aortic aperture lies at the level of (   ).

    A. 6th thoracic vertebra

    B. 8th thoracic vertebra

    C. 10th thoracic vertebra

    D. 12th thoracic vertebra

23. The esophageal aperture lies at the level of (   ).

    A. 6th thoracic vertebra

    B. 8th thoracic vertebra

    C. 10th thoracic vertebra

    D. 12th thoracic vertebra

24. The vena cava aperture lies at the level of (   ).

    A. 6th thoracic vertebra

    B. 8th thoracic vertebra

    C. 10th thoracic vertebra

    D. 12th thoracic vertebra

25. About the obliquus externus abdominis, which of the statements is **wrong**? (   )

    A. It is the most superficial muscle of anterolateral group muscles of abdomen.

    B. The muscle fibers radiate downward, forward and medially.

    C. Its aponeurosis forms the posterior layer of sheath of the rectus abdominis.

    D. It takes part in respiration.

26. The inguinal ligament is formed by (   ).

    A. aponeurosis of obliquus externus abdominis

    B. aponeurosis of obliquus internus abdominis

    C. aponeurosis of transversus abdominis

    D. transverse fascia

27. Obliquus internus abdominis takes part in forming the following structures, **except** (   ).

    A. inguinal ligament

    B. cremaster

    C. inguinal falx

    D. sheath of rectus abdominis

28. Which of the following is the insertion of pectoralis minor? (   )

    A. Coracoid process of scapula

    B. Crest of greater tubercle of humerus

    C. Medial border of scapula

    D. Crest of lesser tubercle of humerus

29. About the sheath of rectus abdominis, which of the statements is **wrong**? (   )

    A. It has anterior and posterior layers.

    B. It is formed by the aponeurosis of three muscles.

    C. Arcuate line is the lateral border of the sheath.

D. The posterior layer of the sheath is absent below arcuate line.

30. Which of the following is **not** associated with the movements of shoulder joint?
   (   )
   A. Pectoralis major
   B. Deltoid
   C. Coracobrachialis
   D. Serratus anterior

31. Which of the following is **not** the muscle of shoulder? (   )
   A. Pectoralis major
   B. Deltoid
   C. Supraspinatus
   D. Teres minor

32. The teres major makes the arm do the following movements, **except** (   ).
   A. abduction
   B. adduction
   C. extension
   D. medial rotation

33. Which of the following does **not** form the shoulder cuff? (   )
   A. Supraspinatus
   B. Infraspinatus
   C. Teres major
   D. Teres minor

34. Which muscle can make the shoulder joint flex and extend? (   )
   A. Pectoralis major
   B. Deltoid
   C. Supraspinatus
   D. Teres major

35. Which of the following can abduct the shoulder joint? (   )
   A. Deltoid and infraspinatus
   B. Deltoid and supraspinatus
   C. infraspinatus and latissimus dorsi
   D. Teres major and deltoid

36. The muscle which flexes both of the shoulder and elbow joints is (   ).
   A. biceps brachii
   B. pectoralis major
   C. latissimus dorsi
   D. deltoid

37. Which of the following is **not** attached to the coracoid process of scapula? (   )
   A. Long head of biceps brachii

B. Short head of biceps brachii

C. Pectoralis minor

D. Coracobrachialis

38. Which of the following is **not** the anterior group of muscles of arm? (   )

A. Biceps brachii

B. Triceps brachii

C. Brachialis

D. Coracobrachialis

39. About the insertion of muscles, which of the statements is **wrong**? (   )

A. Biceps brachii is inserted to the tuberosity of ulna.

B. Triceps brachii is inserted to the olecranon of ulna.

C. Brachialis is inserted to the tuberosity of ulna.

D. Coracobrachialis is inserted to the middle part of humerus.

40. Which of the structures passes through the articular capsule of shoulder joint?

(   )

A. Tendon of biceps brachii

B. Tendon of triceps brachii

C. Tendon of brachialis

D. Tendon of coracobrachialis

41. Which of the following is **not** the anterior group of muscle of forearm? (   )

A. Brachioradialis

B. Pronator teres

C. Palmaris longus

D. Supinator

42. Which of the muscles can flex the wrist joint? (   )

A. Brachioradialis

B. Pronator teres

C. Palmaris longus

D. Supinator

43. Which of the muscles can extend the elbow joint? (   )

A. Brachioradialis

B. Biceps brachii

C. Brachialis

D. Triceps brachii

44. About the iliopsoas, which of the statements is **wrong**? (   )

A. It is formed by psoas major and iliacus.

B. It is inserted into the greater trochanter of femur.

C. It is the most powerful flexor of the thigh.

D. It also can rotate the thigh laterally.

45. The muscle which flexes both of the hip joint and knee joint is (   ).
    A. quadriceps femoris
    B. biceps femoris
    C. sartorius
    D. adductor longus

46. Which of the following belongs to the medial group of muscles of the thigh? (   )
    A. Semitendinosus
    B. Biceps femoris
    C. Gracilis
    D. Sartorius

47. Which of the muscles can extend the hip joint? (   )
    A. Iliopsoas
    B. Sartorius
    C. Gracilis
    D. Gluteus maximus

48. About the medial group of muscles of thigh, which of the statements is **wrong**?
    (   )
    A. It consists of five muscles.
    B. It lies on the lateral side of the thigh.
    C. All of the muscles arise near the obturator foramen.
    D. It can adduct, flex and laterally rotate the thigh.

49. Which of the following does **not** belong to the muscles of pelvic girdle? (   )
    A. Iliopsoas
    B. Pectineus
    C. Tensor fasciae latae
    D. Piriformis

50. Which muscle passes through the greater sciatic foramen? (   )
    A. Gluteus maximus
    B. Gluteus medius
    C. Gluteus minimus
    D. Piriformis

51. About the gluteus maximus, which of the statements is **wrong**? (   )
    A. It arises from the dorsal portion of iliac ala, dorsal surface of sacrum and coc-
       cyx, and sacrotuberous ligament.
    B. It is inserted into the iliotibial tract and gluteal tuberosity of the femur.
    C. It is a powerful flexor of the thigh.
    D. It is a powerful lateral rotator of the thigh.

52. Which of the following belongs to the anterior group of muscles of the leg? (   )
    A. Gastrocnemius

    B. Peroneus longus

    C. Extensor hallucis longus

    D. Soleus

53. Which of the following belongs to the posterior group of muscles of the leg? (　　)

    A. Flexor digitorum longus

    B. Peroneus longus

    C. Tibialis anterior

    D. Extensor digitorum longus

54. Which of the following belongs to the lateral group of muscles of the leg? (　　)

    A. Tibialis posterior

    B. Peroneus brevis

    C. Tibialis anterior

    D. Extensor digitorum longus

55. The muscle which can flex the knee joint is (　　).

    A. tibialis posterior

    B. gastrocnemius

    C. tibialis anterior

    D. quadriceps femoris

56. About the biceps femoris, which of the statements is **wrong**? (　　)

    A. It lies laterally on the back of the thigh.

    B. It has two heads of origin.

    C. Long head arises from the ischial tuberosity.

    D. Short head arises from the ischial tuberosity.

57. Which muscle can plantar-flex and evert the ankle joint? (　　)

    A. Extensor digitorum longus

    B. Peroneus longus

    C. Tibialis anterior

    D. Tibialis posterior

58. Which muscle can dorsiflex and invert the ankle joint? (　　)

    A. Extensor digitorum longus

    B. Peroneus longus

    C. Tibialis anterior

    D. Tibialis posterior

59. About the triceps surae, which of the statements is right? (　　)

    A. It belongs to the deep layer muscle of the leg.

    B. It consists of the gastrocnemius, soleus and plantaris.

    C. It is inserted into the posterior surface of the calcaneus bone.

    D. It can dorsiflex the ankle joint.

60. Which of the following belongs to the muscles of shoulder? (　　)

A. Pectoralis major

B. Pectoralis major

C. Latissimus dorsi

D. Deltoid

Ⅱ. Double choices (Choose the two best answers among the following choices, and write down the corresponding letters in bracket)

1. Which ones of the following do **not** belong to the supplementary structures of skeletal muscles? (   )

   A. Tendon

   B. Fascia

   C. Synovial bursa

   D. Aponeurosis

   E. Retinaculum

2. The structures passing through the aortic hiatus are (   ).

   A. esophagus

   B. abdominal aorta

   C. anterior and posterior vagal trunks

   D. inferior vena cava

   E. thoracic duct

3. The structures passing through the esophageal hiatus are (   ).

   A. esophagus

   B. abdominal aorta

   C. anterior and posterior vagal trunks

   D. inferior vena cava

   E. thoracic duct

4. Which ones of the following can elevate the mandible? (   )

   A. Mylohyoid

   B. Lateral pterygoid

   C. Temporalis

   D. Masseter

   E. Digastric

5. Which ones of the following can depress the hyoid bone? (   )

   A. Stylohyoid

   B. Geniohyoid

   C. Omohyoid

   D. Masseter

   E. Sternohyoid

6. About the trapezius, which ones of the statements are **wrong**? (   )

A. It is one of the deep muscles of the back.

B. It is responsible for the sloping ridge of the neck.

C. It is inserted into the lateral one third of clavicle, acromion, spine of scapula.

D. Spines of all lumbar vertebrae are a part of the origins of the muscle.

E. It can steady, raise, descend, retract and rotate the scapula.

7. About the latissimus dorsi, which ones of the statements are **wrong**? (   )

A. It belongs to the long muscle.

B. It is one of the superficial muscles of the back.

C. It arises from the spines of the lower thoracic vertebrae, thoracolumbar fascia, and iliac crest.

D. It is inserted into the floor of intertubercular sulcus.

E. It can extend, abduct and laterally rotates the humerus.

8. The muscles which can invert the foot are (   ).

A. gastrocnemius

B. peroneus longus

C. extensor hallucis longus

D. tibialis anterior

E. tibialis posterior

9. Which ones of the muscles belong to the extrinsic muscles of thorax? (   )

A. Pectoralis major

B. Deltoid

C. Coracobrachialis

D. Serratus anterior

E. Biceps brachii

10. Which ones of the following are **not** the formation of obliquus externus abdominis?
(   )

A. Inguinal ligament

B. Cremaster

C. Inguinal falx

D. Superficial inguinal ring

E. Linea alba

11. The muscles which can flex the knee joint are (   ).

A. quadriceps femoris

B. biceps femoris

C. sartorius

D. adductor longus

E. gracilis

12. Which ones of the following belong to the posterior group of muscles of the thigh?
(   )

    A. Semitendinosus

    B. Biceps femoris

    C. Gracilis

    D. Sartorius

    E. Quadriceps femoris

13. About the pectoralis minor, which ones of the statements are right? (　　)

    A. It lies deep to the serratus anterior

    B. It arises from the upper six costal cartilages.

    C. It is inserted into the coracoid process of scapula.

    D. It can draw the scapula backward and downward.

    E. When the scapula is fixed, it helps the inspiration.

14. The muscles which can both extend the hip joint and flex the knee joint are (　　).

    A. quadriceps femoris

    B. biceps femoris

    C. sartorius

    D. adductor longus

    E. semimembranosus

15. Which ones of the following belong to the anterior group of muscles of the leg?

    (　　)

    A. Gastrocnemius

    B. Peroneus longus

    C. Extensor hallucis longus

    D. Flexor digitorum longus

    E. Extensor digitorum longus

16. About the rectus abdominis, which ones of the statements are **wrong**? (　　)

    A. It is a long muscle with multiple bellies.

    B. It lies on each side of the linea alba.

    C. It is enclosed by sheath of rectus abdominis.

    D. The posterior layer of the sheath is absent above arcuate line.

    E. It can move the vertebral column in extension and rotation.

17. About the biceps brachii, which ones of the statements are **wrong**? (　　)

    A. It has two heads.

    B. Long head arises from the coracoid process.

    C. Short head arises from the supraglenoid tubercle.

    D. It is inserted into the tuberosity of radius.

    E. It can flex the shoulder and elbow joints, supinate forearm.

18. About the quadriceps femoris, which ones of the statements are **wrong**? (　　)

    A. It lies in front surface of the thigh.

    B. It is the largest muscle of the body.

C. It consists of four muscles.

D. Each of the muscles arises from the linea aspera.

E. It is the only flexor of the leg.

19. Which ones of the muscles can flex the wrist joint? (   )

   A. Brachioradialis

   B. Pronator teres

   C. Palmaris longus

   D. Supinator

   E. Flexor carpi radialis

20. About the deltoid, which ones of the statements are right? (   )

   A. It belongs to the muscles of arm.

   B. It forms the rounded contour of the shoulder.

   C. It arises from the coracoid process.

   D. It is inserted into the deltoid tuberosity of humerus.

   E. It is the most powerful adductor of the arm.

III. Fill the blanks (Fill the most appropriate words in the blanks)

1. According to the shape, muscles are divided into four types, _____, _____, _____ and _____.

2. The supplementary structures of skeletal muscles consist of _____, ———, _____ and _____.

3. The masticatory muscles consist of _____, _____, _____ and _____.

4. The superficial muscles in the neck include _____ and _____.

5. The anterior group of muscles of the thigh include _____ and _____.

6. Three openings in the diaphragm are _____, _____ and _____.

7. The suprahyoid muscles include _____, _____, _____ and _____.

8. The infrahyoid muscles include _____, _____, _____ and _____.

9. Below arcuate line, the anterior layer of sheath of rectus abdominis is formed by the aponeuroses of _____, _____ and _____.

10. The extrinsic muscles of thorax consist of _____, _____, and _____.

11. Triceps surae is formed by _____ and _____.

12. Two heads of the biceps brachii arise from _____ and _____, respectively.

13. Shoulder cuff is formed by the tendons of _____, _____, _____ and _____.

14. Anterior group of muscles of arm includes _____, _____, and _____.

15. The muscles which can flex the interphalangeal joints of medial four fingers are _____ and _____.

16. Iliopsoas is composed of two muscles, _____ and _____.

17. Quadriceps femoris consists of 4 muscles, _____ , _____ , _____ and _____.

18. Medial group of muscles of the thigh contains _____ , _____ , _____ , _____ and _____.

19. The muscle which can flex the hip and knee joints is _____.

20. The structures passing through the aortic hiatus are _____ and _____.

IV. Answer questions briefly

1. Please describe the openings in the diaphragm as well as the organs transmitting them.

2. Please describe the groups, names and main functions of the muscles of the thigh.

3. Please describe the names and functions of the masticatory muscles.

4. Please describe the location, origin and insertion, function of the sternocleidomastoid.

5. Please describe the location, origin and insertion, function of the biceps brachii.

6. Please describe the location, origin and insertion, function of the gluteus maximus.

7. Please describe the formation of the sheath of rectus abdominis.

8. Please describe the location, origin and insertion, function of the quadriceps femoris.

9. Please describe the location, origin and insertion, function of the deltoid.

10. Please describe the groups, names and main functions of the muscles of the arm.

V. Answer questions in detail

1. Please describe the muscles moving the shoulder joint.

2. Please describe the muscles moving the elbow joint.

3. Please describe the muscles moving the hip joint.

4. Please describe the muscles moving the knee joint.

VI. Problems in life

What causes "rigor mortis"?

Part 2 Splanchnology

Chapter 4   The General Description

I. **Single choice (Choose the best answer among the following four choices, and write down the corresponding letter in bracket)**

1. Which of the following belongs to the parenchymatous organ? (   )
   A. Stomach
   B. Esophagus
   C. Bronchus
   D. Lung

2. Which of the following is the most inner structure in the tubular organ wall? (   )
   A. Mucosa
   B. Submucosa
   C. Muscular layer
   D. Serosa

3. Which of the following structures has a "hilum"? (   )
   A. Stomach
   B. Spleen
   C. Esophagus
   D. Jejunum

4. According to the nine regions of human abdomen, which of the following is just single region? (   )
   A. Hypochondriac region
   B. Lumbar region
   C. Iliac region
   D. Epigastric region

5. Which of the following is the transverse plane that divides the abdomen into four regions? (   )
   A. Trans-pyloric line
   B. The approximately pass through umbilicus line
   C. Midaxillary line

D. Midclavicular line

II. Double choices (Choose the best two answers among the following choices, and write down the corresponding letters in bracket)

1. Which ones of the following do **not** belong to systems in splanchnology? (　　)

   A. Circulation system

   B. Respiratory system

   C. Reproductive system

   D. Alimentary system

   E. Endocrine system

2. According to the structure and morphology of visceral organs, it may be classified as two different types of organ, including (　　).

   A. lobular organ

   B. tubular organ

   C. parenchymal organ

   D. fibrous organ

   E. compact organ

3. Which ones of the following possess "hilum" structure? (　　)

   A. Liver

   B. Lung

   C. Duodena

   D. Ileum

   E. Rectum

4. Which ones of the following are the transverse plane that divides the abdomen into nine regions? (　　)

   A. Trans-pyloric plane

   B. The approximately pass through umbilicus plane.

   C. Midaxillary plane

   D. Subcostal plane

   E. Trans-tubercular plane

5. According nine regions of human abdomen, which ones of the following are single regions? (　　)

   A. Hypochondriac region

   B. Lumbar region

   C. Iliac region

   D. Epigastric region

   E. Pubic region

Chapter 5　The Alimentary System

Ⅰ. **Single choice（Choose the best answer among the following four choices, and write down the corresponding letter in bracket）**

1. There are communications between the vestibule of the mouth and the proper oral cavity, which locate in （　　）.
   A. oral lips
   B. cheeks
   C. aperture behind the third molar teeth
   D. oral fissure

2. Which of the following is the internal boundary of the vestibular of the mouth?
   （　　）
   A. Oral lips
   D. Cheeks
   C. Gums and teeth
   D. Palate

3. Which of the following is the roof of the oral cavity proper? （　　）
   A. Oral lips
   B. Cheeks
   C. Gums and teeth
   D. Palate

4. The boundary between the proper oral cavity and the oral pharyngeal cavity is usually termed （　　）.
   A. pharyngeal isthmus
   B. hard palate
   C. soft palate
   D. root of tongue

5. Where is the opening of parotid duct? （　　）
   A. On inside of cheeks opposite the upper second molar tooth
   B. On inside of cheeks opposite the lower second molar tooth
   C. On inside of cheeks opposite the upper first molar tooth
   D. On inside of cheeks opposite the lower first molar tooth

6. How much proportion does the soft palate hold in the whole palate? （　　）
   A. Posterior two third
   B. Posterior one third
   C. Posterior two fifth

D. Posterior one fifth

7. Which of the following contains the palatine tonsil? (　　)

A. Tongue surface

B. Cheek surface

C. Nasopharyngeal surface

D. Tonsil fossa

8. According to the formation of the isthmus of fauces, which of the following does **not** involve in? (　　)

A. Uvula

B. Root of tongue

C. Palatopharyngeal arch

D. Free margin of palatine velum

9. Which of the following does **not** belong to the periodontal structures? (　　)

A. Gums

B. Sockets of the alveolar

C. Periodontal membrane

D. Dental pulp

10. Which of the following does **not** belong to the dental elements? (　　)

A. Dentine

B. Enamel

C. Cement

D. Dental pulp

11. Which of the following is the structure that makes up the dental pulp? (　　)

A. Dentine

B. Enamel

C. Cement

D. Vessels and nerves

12. Which of the following is the boundary between the oral part and the pharyngeal part of tongue? (　　)

A. Root of tongue

B. Apex of tongue

C. Terminal sulcus

D. Body of tongue

13. Which of the following is near to the terminal sulcus of tongue? (　　)

A. Vallate papillae

B. Fungiform papillae

C. Filiform papillae

D. Foliate papillae

14. Taste buds are usually found on the papillae, which of the following does **not** have

the taste buds? (   )

A. Vallate papillae

B. Fungiform papillae

C. Filiform papillae

D. Foliate papillae

15. Which muscle mainly helps to protrude the tongue? (   )

A. Genioglossus

B. Hyoglossus

C. Styloglossus

D. Mylohyoid muscle

16. What is the opening for the parotid duct? (   )

A. Sublingual caruncle

B. Papilla of parotid duct

C. Palate

D. Pharynx

17. Which of the following is where the submandibular gland opening locates? (   )

A. Sublingual caruncle

B. Papilla of parotid duct

C. Palate

D. Pharynx

18. Which one is the upper boundary of the pharynx? (   )

A. Soft palate

B. Base of skull

C. Atlas

D. Axis

19. The lower boundary of the pharynx is (   ).

A. atlas

B. axis

C. the fifth cervical vertebra

D. the sixth cervical vertebra

20. Which of the following locates behind the tubal torus? (   )

A. Pharyngeal recess

B. Tonsil fossa

C. Pharyngeal isthmus

D. Choanae

21. The following structures locate in the laryngopharynx, **except** (   ).

A. pharyngeal recess

B. tonsillar ring

C. piriform recess

D. tonsil fossa

22. Which of the following is the landmark that separates the esophagus from the pharynx? (   )

A. The sixth cervical vertebra

B. The fifth cervical vertebra

C. The fourth cervical vertebra

D. The third cervical vertebra

23. Which of the following is the shortest part of the esophagus? (   )

A. Cervical part

B. Thoracic part

C. Abdominal part

D. Pelvic part

24. About three constrictions in the whole esophagus, how long is the distance between
the second constriction to the incisor teeth? (   )

A. 15 cm

B. 25 cm

C. 35 cm

D. 45 cm

25. The following are the relative locations of the esophagus constrictions, **except**
(   ).

A. the sixth cervical vertebra

B. the fourth thoracic vertebra

C. the tenth thoracic vertebra

D. the twelfth thoracic vertebra

26. The entrance of the stomach is termed (   ).

A. pyloric orifice

B. cardiac orifice

C. pyloric canal

D. pyloric antrum

27. Which of the following is the largest part of the stomach? (   )

A. Cardiac part

B. Fundus of stomach

C. Body of stomach

D. Pyloric stomach

28. Which of the following is the landmark that separates the body of stomach from the
pyloric part? (   )

A. Angular incisure

B. Great curvature

C. Pyloric orifice

    D. Cardiac orifice

29. The outlet of the stomach is termed (   ).

    A. pyloric orifice

    B. cardiac orifice

    C. pyloric canal

    D. pyloric antrum

30. Which of the following is the landmark that separates the pyloric antrum from the pyloric canal? (   )

    A. Angular incisure

    B. Great curvature

    C. Lesser curvature

    D. Intermediate groove

31. Which of the following is the relative location of the cardiac orifice? (   )

    A. The fourth cervical vertebra

    B. The tenth thoracic vertebra

    C. The eleventh thoracic vertebra

    D. The twelfth thoracic vertebra

32. Which of the following is the relative location of the pyloric orifice? (   )

    A. The tenth thoracic vertebra

    B. The eleventh thoracic vertebra

    C. The twelfth thoracic vertebra

    D. The first lumbar vertebra

33. The following are **not** the adjacent organs of the left part of the anterior surface of stomach, **except** (   ).

    A. base of left lung

    B. left pleura

    C. left lobe of liver

    D. spleen

34. The following forms the stomach bed, **except** (   ).

    A. left suprarenal gland

    B. upper part of left kidney

    C. pancreas

    D. liver

35. Which one forms the pyloric sphincter? (   )

    A. Mucosa layer of stomach

    B. Muscular layer of stomach

    C. Submucosa layer of stomach

    D. Peritoneum layer of stomach

36. Which of the following is the outmost layer of the gastric wall? (   )

    A. Mucosa layer of stomach

    B. Muscular layer of stomach

    C. Submucosa layer of stomach

    D. Peritoneum layer of stomach

37. The shortest part of the duodenum is (　　).

    A. superior part of duodenum

    B. descending part of duodenum

    C. horizontal part of duodenum

    D. ascending part of duodenum

38. Which of the following is the relative location of ascending part of duodenum?
    (　　)

    A. The level of the tenth thoracic vertebra

    B. The level of the eleventh thoracic vertebra

    C. The level of the twelfth thoracic vertebra

    D. The level of the second lumbar vertebra

39. Which of the following contains the major duodenal papilla? (　　)

    A. Superior part of duodenum

    B. Descending part of duodenum

    C. Horizontal part of duodenum

    D. Ascending part of duodenum

40. Which of the following is the unique feature of jejunum compared with ileum?
    (　　)

    A. Almost absence in the aggregated lymphatic follicles.

    B. Lower part of jejunum locates in the pelvic cavity.

    C. A few circular folds present in the upper part of jejunum.

    D. The jejunum walls are thicker than ileum's.

41. Which of the following is the unique feature of large intestine compared with small
    intestine? (　　)

    A. It possesses the largest mesentery.

    B. It possesses three colic bands.

    C. It has a smaller calibre.

    D. Most parts are free in position.

42. According to the unique features of large intestine, which of the following is **not**
    true? (　　)

    A. Colic bands

    B. Haustra of colon

    C. Epiploic appendices

    D. Mesentery

43. According to the defining the McBurney's point, which of the following is true?

(   )

  A. The junction of the lateral one third and middle one third line between the right anterior superior iliac spine and the umbilicus.

  B. The junction of the internal one third and middle one third line between the right anterior superior iliac spine and the umbilicus.

  C. The junction of the lateral two third and internal one third line between the right anterior superior iliac spine and the umbilicus.

  D. The junction of the lateral one third and middle two third line between the right anterior superior iliac spine and the umbilicus.

44. Which of the following continues with the cecum? (   )

  A. Ascending colon

  B. Transverse colon

  C. Descending colon

  ·D. Sigmoid colon

45. The longest part of the colon is (   ).

  A. ascending colon

  B. transverse colon

  C. descending colon

  D. sigmoid colon

46. Which of the following is the level at which sigmoid continues with the rectum? (   )

  A. The fifth lumbar vertebrae

  B. The first sacral vertebrae

  C. The second sacral vertebrae

  D. The third sacral vertebrae

47. Which of the following is the direction of the rectum sacral flexure? (   )

  A. Left to right

  B. Anteroposterior

  C. Upper to lower

  D. Right to left

48. What portion of the rectum is totally surrounded by the peritoneum? (   )

  A. The upper 1/3 of the rectum

  B. The upper 2/3 of the rectum

  C. The lower 1/3 of the rectum

  D. The lower 2/3 of the rectum

49. The structure formed by the peritoneum between the rectum and urinary bladder is termed (   ).

  A. rectouterine pouch

  B. rectovesical pouch

C. retrocecal recess

D. hepatorenal recess

50. The terminology defined the vertical mucous folds in the lower part of anal canal is the (   ).

A. anal valves

B. anal sinus

C. anal pecten

D. anal columns

51. Which of the following involves in the formation of anal sinus? (   )

A. Anal valves

B. White line

C. Anal pecten

D. Dentate line

52. What separates the anal mucous membrane with the anal skin? (   )

A. Anal sinus

B. White line

C. Anal pecten

D. Dentate line

53. Which of the following is the marking that separates the subcutaneous part of the external sphincter from the lower part of the internal sphincter? (   )

A. Anal valves

B. White line

C. Anal pecten

D. Dentate line

54. Which of the following is the largest single gland in human body? (   )

A. Parotid gland

B. Sublingual gland

C. Salivary gland

D. Liver

55. The followings are the salivary glands, **except** (   ).

A. parotid gland

B. sublingual gland

C. salivary gland

D. liver

56. According to the space occupied by the most part of liver in the normal condition, which one is correct? (   )

A. Left hypochondriac space

B. Epigastric space

C. Right hypochondriac space

D. Umbilical space

57. Which of the following is the ligament separated the liver into right lobe and left lobe on the diaphragmatic surface? (   )

A. Hepatic round ligament

B. Coronary ligament

C. Triangular ligament

D. Falciform ligament

58. The structure located anterior to the porta hepatis is the (   ).

A. right hepatic lobe

B. left hepatic lobe

C. caudate lobe

D. quadrate lobe

59. The following are the impressions on the visceral surface of liver made by the others organs, **except** (   ).

A. left kidney

B. stomach

C. gallbladder

D. right colic flexure

60. Which of the following is the terminology defined the union of sulcus for the inferior vena cava and the fossa for gallbladder? (   )

A. The left longitudinal groove

B. The right longitudinal groove

C. The fissure for the hepatic round ligament

D. Coronary groove

61. Which of the following is the terminology defined the union of fissure for the ligamentum venosum and the ligamentum teres hepatic? (   )

A. The left longitudinal groove

B. The right longitudinal groove

C. The fissure for the hepatic round ligament

D. Coronary groove

62. Which of the following is the ligament involved in the fibrous cord homologous to the fetus umbilicus vein? (   )

A. Hepatic round ligament

B. Coronary ligament

C. Triangular ligament

D. Falciform ligament

63. The following statements about the porta hepatis, which one is correct? (   )

A. It locates on the diaphragmatic surface of liver.

B. It is an entrance of all structures entering into or leaving out liver.

C. It is an extremely narrow cleft.

D. It contains the portal vein.

64. Which of the following is the rightest structure in lesser oment? (   )

A. Portal vein

B. Hepatic arteries

C. Common hepatic ducts

D. Bile duct

65. Which of the following is the organ that produce the bile? (   )

A. Gallbladder

B. Small intestine

C. Pancreas

D. Liver

66. The left and right hepatic duct joins together to form (   ).

A. cystic duct

B. common bile duct

C. common hepatic duct

D. hepatic ducts

67. Which of the following is the structure which joins with the cystic duct to form the common the bile duct? (   )

A. Left hepatic duct

B. Right hepatic duct

C. Bile neck

D. Common hepatic duct

68. Which of the following is the opening location of the hepatopancreatic ampulla? (   )

A. Superior portion of duodenum

B. Descending portion of duodenum

C. Horizontal portion of duodenum

D. Ascending portion of duodenum

69. Which of the following is **not** the partition of pancreas? (   )

A. Head

B. Fundus

C. Neck

D. Tail

70. Which of the following is the organ that secretes the insulin? (   )

A. Liver

B. Parotid

C. Sublingual gland

D. Pancreas

II. Double choices(Choose the two best answers among the following choices, and write down the corresponding letters in bracket)

1. Which ones of glands do **not** belong to the salivary gland? (   )
   A. Parotid
   B. Sublingual gland
   C. Submandibular gland
   D. Pancreas
   E. Liver

2. Which ones of the following consist mainly of muscle covered by the skin and mucous membrane? (   )
   A. Lips
   B. Tongue
   C. Pharynx
   D. Larynx
   E. Cheeks

3. Which ones of the following consist of not only the roof of mouth, but also the floor of nasal cavity? (   )
   A. Mandible
   B. Tongue
   C. Hard palatine
   D. Soft palatine
   E. Cheeks

4. Which ones of the following involve in the formation of the isthmus of fauces?
   (   )
   A. Hard palatine
   B. Uvula
   C. Palatopharyngeal arch
   D. Palatoglossal arch
   E. Epiglottis

5. The tongue is differed into two parts by the terminal sulcus, these parts are (   ).
   A. body of the tongue
   B. apex of the tongue
   C. root of the tongue
   D. dorsum of the tongue
   E. inferior surface of the tongue

6. Which ones of the following belong to the extrinsic lingual muscles? (   )
   A. Genioglossus
   B. Mylohyoid
   C. Styloglossus

　　D. Omohyoid

　　E. Sternohyoideus

7. Which ones of the following belong to the structures of the nasopharynx? (　　)

　　A. Tonsil fossa

　　B. Tubal torus

　　C. Piriform recess

　　D. Pharyngeal recess

　　E. Epiglottis fossa

8. Which ones of the following are the structures behind the oropharynx? (　　)

　　A. Atlas

　　B. Axis

　　C. The third cervical vertebrae

　　D. The fourth cervical vertebrae

　　E. The fifth cervical vertebrae

9. Which ones of the following are the marking of the becoming the esophagus from the pharynx? (　　)

　　A. Lower board of the cricoid cartilage

　　B. The sixth cervical vertebrae

　　C. Thyroid cartilage

　　D. The first thoracic vertebrae

　　E. The first tracheal cartilage ring

10. Which ones of the following are the organs that have the location contact with the right half of stomach? (　　)

　　A. Right kidney

　　B. Right suprarenal gland

　　C. Decum

　　D. Left liver lobe

　　E. Quadrate lobe

11. The following are the structure features of the descending part of duodenum, **except** (　　).

　　A. major duodenum papilla

　　B. pylorus valve

　　C. minor duodenum papilla

　　D. ileocecal valve

　　E. ligament of treitz

12. The following are the features of the jejunum, **except** (　　).

　　A. thinner wall

　　B. few circular folds

　　C. shorter in length

D. more villus

E. aggregated lymphatic follicles

13. Which ones of the following connect with the posterior abdominal wall by the mesentery? (   )

A. Stomach

B. Liver

C. Duodenum

D. Jejunum

E. Ileum

14. Which ones of the following have the relative unmoved location in abdominal cavity? (   )

A. Cecum

B. Ascending colon

C. Transverse colon

D. Descending colon

E. Sigmoid colon

15. Which ones of the following have the mesocolon? (   )

A. Cecum

B. Ascending colon

C. Transverse colon

D. Descending colon

E. Sigmoid colon

16. Which ones of the following are the features of the rectum? (   )

A. Right colic flexure

B. Left colic flexure

C. Sacral flexure

D. Perineal flexure

E. Mesocolon

17. Which ones of the following are located in front of the rectum? (   )

A. Urinary bladder

B. Vagina

C. Sacrum

D. Coccyx

E. Ovary

18. Which ones of the following involves in the formation of anal sinus? (   )

A. Dentate line

B. Anal valves

C. Anal pecten

D. White line

E. Anal columns

19. Which ones of the following are the hepatic surfaces? (　　)

A. Anterior surface

B. Lateral surface

C. Posterior surface

D. Visceral surface

E. Diaphragmatic surface

20. The structures located anterior or posterior to the porta hepatis in the normal condition are (　　).

A. right lobe

B. left lobe

C. quadrate lobe

D. caudate lobe

E. the fossa for the vena cava

21. Which ones of the following form the right longitudinal groove on the hepatic visceral surface? (　　)

A. Fissure for the ligamentum venosum

B. Sulcus for the inferior vena cava

C. Fossa for the gallbladder

D. Fissure for the ligamentum teres hepatis

E. Porta hepatic

22. Which ones of the following form the left longitudinal groove on the hepatic visceral surface? (　　)

A. Fissure for the ligamentum venosum

B. Sulcus for the inferior vena cava

C. Fossa for the gallbladder

D. Fissure for the ligamentum teres hepatis

E. Porta hepatis

23. Which ones of the following belong to the structure of liver on the diaphragmatic surface? (　　)

A. Bare area

B. Sulcus for the inferior vena cava

C. Fossa for the gallbladder

D. Porta hepatis

E. Galciform ligament

24. Which ones of the following connect with the porta hepatis by the lesser omentum? (　　)

A. Great curvature of stomach

B. Lesser curvature of stomach

  C. Cardiac part of stomach

  D. The first part of duodenum

  E. The second part of duodenum

25. Which ones of the following are ducts that form the common hepatic duct? (　　)

  A. Cystic duct

  B. Common bile duct

  C. Left hepatic duct

  D. Right hepatic duct

  E. Segmental bile duct

26. Which ones of the following open directly into the descending part of duodenum? (　　)

  A. Cystic duct

  B. Common bile duct

  C. Left hepatic duct

  D. Right hepatic duct

  E. Pancreatic duct

27. Which ones of the following are located anterior to the epiploic foramen? (　　)

  A. Inferior vena cava

  B. Porta vein

  C. Common bile duct

  D. Quadrate lobe

  E. Left lobe

28. Which ones of the following are the vessels that enter into the liver in the normal condition? (　　)

  A. Left hepatic vein

  B. Right hepatic vein

  C. Middle hepatic vein

  D. Porta vein

  E. Proper hepatic artery

29. On the hepatic diaphragmatic surface, the liver can be divided into (　　).

  A. left lobe

  B. right lobe

  C. quadrate lobe

  D. caudate lobe

  E. lingual lobe

30. Which ones of the following are the function of the pancreas? (　　)

  A. Releasing the digestive enzymes

  B. Sorbing the nutrition

  C. Secreting the insulin

    D. Swallowing the food

    E. Chewing the food

Ⅲ. Fill the blanks (Fill the most appropriate words in the blanks)

1. The alimentary system consists of _____ and _____.

2. The salivary glands include _____, _____ and _____.

3. The digestive gland with the digestive and endocrine function is _____.

4. The parotid duct opening on the inside cheeks locates _____.

5. The palatine consists of two portions including the anterior _____ hard palatine and the posterior _____ soft palatine.

6. The tonsil fossa contains _____.

7. All teeth have a similar basic structure including _____, _____ and _____.

8. The teeth elements consist of _____, _____ and _____.

9. The periodontal membrane is formed by the _____.

10. The papillae on the tongue have four types including _____, _____, _____ and _____.

11. The tongue includes _____, _____ and _____ three parts.

12. In the nasopharynx, the prominence behind the pharyngeal opening of auditory tube is termed _____, behind which lies the _____.

13. The boundary between the oral cavity and oropharynx is _____.

14. The boundary between the nasopharynx and oropharynx is _____.

15. The boundary between the oropharynx and laryngopharynx is _____.

16. The boundary between the laryngopharynx and esophagus is _____.

17. The piriform recesses locate at _____.

18. The stomach is divided into four parts including _____, _____, _____ and _____.

19. The cardiac orifice locates at the level of the _____ thoracic vertebrae, and the pyloric orifice locates at the level of lower board of the _____ lumbar vertebrae.

20. The structure that separates the body of stomach with the pyloric part of stomach is _____, and the structure that separates the pyloric sinus from the pyloric canal is _____.

21. The structure of the gastric wall consists of _____, _____, _____ and _____.

22. The stomach has two openings termed _____ and _____.

23. The duodenum is divided into four parts including _____, _____, _____ and _____.

24. The opening of the hepatopancreatic ampulla is _____; the opening of the ac-

cessory pancreatic duct is _____.

25. The most unique structure features of the large intestine include _____, _____ and _____.

26. The large intestine includes _____, _____, _____, _____ and _____.

27. The rectum possesses two curves known as _____ and _____.

28. The peritoneum between the urinary bladder and rectum reflects to form _____, and between the vagina and rectum reflects to form _____.

29. The anal sinus is formed by _____ and _____.

30. The landmark structure that separates the anal mucous membrane from anal skin is _____.

31. The liver lobes includes _____, _____, _____ and _____.

32. The right longitudinal groove of liver is formed by the _____ and _____.

33. The left longitudinal groove of liver is formed by the _____ and _____.

34. The ligaments attaching with liver are _____, _____, _____, _____ and _____.

35. The liver has two surfaces including _____ and _____.

36. On the hepatic superior surface, the area which is not covered by peritoneum terms _____.

37. The structure that transmits the porta hepatis includes _____, _____, _____, _____ and _____.

38. The left and right hepatic duct join together to form _____, which unites with the cystic duct to form _____.

39. The gallbladder is divided four parts including _____, _____, _____ and _____.

40. The pancreas is divided four parts including _____, _____, _____ and _____.

IV. Answer questions briefly

1. Please describe the basic structure and composition of tooth.
2. Please describe the location of the pharynx.
3. Please describe the structure of the nasopharynx.
4. Please describe the composition of tonsil ring.
5. Please describe the partitions of stomach.
6. Please describe the composition of small intestine.
7. Please describe the partitions of duodenum.
8. Please describe the composition of the large intestine.
9. Please describe the common structure character of large intestine.
10. Please describe the projection on the body surface marking for the vermiform appen-

dix base.

11. Please describe the structure of anal canal.

12. Please describe the anatomic division of liver lobes.

13. Please describe the formation of biliary ducts outside liver.

14. Please describe the partitions of the pancreas.

15. Please describe the partitions of gallbladder.

V. Answer questions in detail

1. Please describe the partitions and structure of the pharynx.

2. Please describe the shape, partitions and position of the stomach.

3. Please describe the shape, partitions and position of the liver.

4. Please describe the structure of the rectum.

VI. Problems in life

1. It often occurs after meals or at night, one may feel a burning pain in the middle of his chest, so what has happened in this guy's alimentary system?

2. Someone can be constipated or have diarrhea, or have hard, dry stools on one day and loose watery stools on another, so what causes for the above?

3. Bright red blood in the toilet bowl when you move your bowels could be a sign of hemorrhoids, which is a very common condition. Do you know the anatomic mechanism on hemorrhoids?

Chapter 6 The Respiratory System

I. **Single choice (Choose the best answer among the following four choices, and write down the corresponding letter in bracket)**

1. Which of the following does **not** belong to the upper respiratory tract? (   )
   A. Nose
   B. Oral cavity
   C. Pharynx
   D. Larynx

2. The mucous membrane lining the upper portion of the nasal cavity is called (   ).
   A. olfactory region
   B. little area
   C. Kiesselbach area
   D. ethmoidal sinuses

3. Which of the following does **not** belong to the paranasal sinuses? (   )
   A. Frontal sinus
   B. Maxillary sinus
   C. Inferior sagittal sinus
   D. Ethmoidal sinus

4. Which of the following belongs to the paranasal sinuses that opens into the spheno-ethmoidal recess? (   )
   A. Frontal sinus
   B. Maxillary sinus
   C. Ethmoidal sinus
   D. Sphenoidal sinus

5. Which of the following belongs to the paranasal sinuses that opens in the superior nasal meatus? (   )
   A. Posterior ethmoidal sinus
   B. Maxillary sinus
   C. Anterior ethmoidal sinus
   D. Frontal sinus

6. Which of the following cartilages forms the laryngeal prominence? (   )
   A. Epiglottic cartilage
   B. Cricoid cartilage
   C. Thyroid cartilage
   D. Arytenoid cartilage

7. Paired laryngeal cartilage is (   ).

    A. thyroid cartilage

    B. cricoid cartilage

    C. arytenoid cartilage

    D. epiglottic cartilage

8. The largest laryngeal cartilage is (   ).

    A. epiglottic cartilage

    B. cricoid cartilage

    C. arytenoid cartilage

    D. thyroid cartilage

9. The fissure of glottis lies between the two (   ).

    A. vocal folds

    B. vestibular folds

    C. ventricle of larynx

    D. palatopharyngeal arch

10. Three parts of the laryngeal cavity do **not** include (   ).

    A. laryngeal vestibule

    B. ventricles of larynx

    C. intermedial cavity of larynx

    D. infraglottic cavity

11. The leaf-shaped elastic cartilage is (   ).

    A. cricoid cartilage

    B. arytenoid cartilage

    C. epiglottic cartilage

    D. thyroid cartilage

12. The lower borders of quadrangular membranes form (   ).

    A. cricotracheal ligaments

    B. vestibular ligaments

    C. median cricothyroid ligaments

    D. vocal ligaments

13. The superior borders of conus elasticus form (   ).

    A. median cricothyroid ligaments

    B. vestibular ligaments

    C. median thyrohyoid ligaments

    D. vocal ligaments

14. The movement of cricothyroid joint can relax or tense (   ).

    A. thyrohyoid membrane

    B. vestibular fold

    C. median cricothyroid ligaments

    D. vocal fold

15. The muscles which can open the glottis is (   ).

    A. posterior cricoarytenoid muscle

    B. cricothyroid muscle

    C. oblique arytenoid muscle

    D. thyroarytenoid muscle

16. The muscles which can relax and shorten the vocal fold is (   ).

    A. lateral cricoarytenoid muscle

    B. thyroarytenoid muscle

    C. cricothyroid muscle

    D. transverse arytenoid muscle

17. The structure that continues with the trachea is (   ).

    A. laryngeal vestibule

    B. intermediate cavity of larynx

    C. ventricle of larynx

    D. infraglottic cavity

18. The bifurcation of trachea is located in the level of (   )

    A. manubrium sterni

    B. sternal angle

    C. body of sternum

    D. xiphoid process

19. Foreign object from the trachea usually goes to the (   ).

    A. stomach

    B. ventricle of larynx

    C. right principal bronchus

    D. left principal bronchus

20. Characteristics of the right principal bronchus are (   ).

    A. shorter and wider

    B. longer and finer

    C. shorter and finer

    D. longer and wider

21. The base of lung is also called (   ).

    A. mediastinal surface

    B. medial surface

    C. diaphragmatic surface

    D. costal surface

22. Which of the following extends to about 2 – 3 cm above the level of the clavicle?
    (   )

    A. Root of lung

B. Apex of lung

C. Cardiac notch

D. Pulmonary ligament

23. About the left lung, which statement is correct? (　　)

A. It is shorter than the right one.

B. There is a horizontal fissure.

C. It is divided into superior, middle and inferior lobes.

D. It is divided into superior and inferior lobes.

24. About the right lung, which statement is correct? (　　)

A. There are a horizontal fissure and an oblique fissure.

B. It is longer than the left one.

C. There is a cardiac notch.

D. It is divided into superior and inferior lobes.

25. Cardiac notch lies in (　　).

A. the anterior border of right lung

B. the inferior border of right lung

C. the anterior border of left lung

D. the inferior border of left lung

26. The root of lung does **not** contain (　　).

A. bifurcation of trachea

B. principle bronchus

C. pulmonary artery

D. pulmonary veins

27. Which of the following does **not** belong to the parietal pleura? (　　)

A. Costal pleura

B. Diaphragmatic pleura

C. Mediastinal pleura

D. Pulmonary pleura

28. The structure **without** pleural covering is (　　).

A. the surface of lung

B. the inferior surface of diaphragm

C. the superior surface of diaphram

D. the inner surface of the thorax

29. Which of the following is a double layer pleura below the root of lung? (　　)

A. Falciform ligament

B. Greater omentum

C. Pulmonary ligament

D. Lesser omentum

30. About the pleural cavity, which statement is **wrong**? (　　)

    A. Two pleural cavities are separated from each other by diaphragm.

    B. It is between the parietal and visceral pleurae.

    C. It contains a film of fluid.

    D. It is negative pressure in the pleural cavity.

II. Double choices(Choose the two best answers among the following choices, and write down the corresponding letters in bracket)

1. Which ones of the following belong to the lower respiratory tract? (　　)

    A. Pharynx

    B. Trachea

    C. Larynx

    D. Principal bronchi

    E. Lungs

2. The nasal cavity is divided into (　　).

    A. nasal vestibule

    B. nasal limen

    C. superior nasal meatuses

    D. proper nasal cavity

    E. inferior nasal meatuses

3. The nasal mucous membrane is divided into (　　).

    A. little area

    B. nasal conchae

    C. nasal meatuses

    D. respiratory region

    E. olfactory region

4. Which ones of the following paranasal sinuses do **not** open in the middle nasal meatuses? (　　)

    A. Middle ethmoidal sinuses

    B. Maxillary sinuses

    C. Sphenoidal sinuses

    D. Anterior ethmoidal sinuses

    E. Posterior ethmoidal sinuses

5. Which ones of the following are narrower in the laryngeal cavity? (　　)

    A. Rima vestibuli

    B. Aditus laryngis

    C. Fissure of glottis

    D. End of the larynx

    E. Laryngeal vestibule

6. The laryngeal cavity is divided into three parts by (　　).

    A. vocal folds

    B. vestibular folds

    C. thyroid cartilage

    D. cricoid cartilage

    E. arytenoid cartilage

7. The ventricles of larynx are the lateral expansions between (　　).

    A. laryngeal vestibule

    B. vestibular folds

    C. infraglottic cavity

    D. quadrangular membranes

    E. vocal folds

8. About the cricoid cartilage, which of the descriptions are correct? (　　)

    A. It is half-ring shaped.

    B. It is at the level of third cervical vertebra.

    C. The lamina is behind.

    D. The arch is in front.

    E. The lamina articulates with the epiglottic cartilage.

9. The cricothyroid joint is located between (　　).

    A. the inferior cornu of the thyroid cartilage

    B. the lamina of cricoid cartilage

    C. the arch of cricoid cartilage

    D. the base of the thyroid cartilage

    E. the lateral surface of cricoid cartilage

10. The cricoarytenoid joint is located between (　　).

    A. the inferior cornu of the arytenoid cartilage

    B. the lamina of cricoid cartilage

    C. the base of the arytenoid cartilage

    D. the lateral surface of cricoid cartilage

    E. the arch of cricoid cartilage

11. The muscles which can tense and lengthen the vocal fold are (　　).

    A. cricothyroid muscle

    B. thyroarytenoid muscle

    C. transverse arytenoid muscle

    D. posterior cricoarytenoid muscle

    E. oblique arytenoid

12. Which statements of the following about trachea are true? (　　)

    A. It is behind the esophagus.

    B. It lies in the middle of neck and upper thorax.

    C. It is divides into the right, middle and left principal bronchi.

    D. Lower border is at the level of the xiphoid process.

    E. Upper border is at the level of sixth cervical vertebra.

13. The wall of trachea is composed of (   ).

    A. tracheal cartilage

    B. smooth muscle

    C. cricoid cartilage

    D. skeletal muscle

    E. thyroid cartilage

14. Which ones of the following about carina of trachea are true? (   )

    A. It is a sagittal semilunar ridge.

    B. It can not be seen through bronchoscope.

    C. It is a guide to the larynx.

    D. It is at the beginning of the trachea.

    E. It is inside the bifurcation of trachea.

15. The right lung is divided into three lobes by (   ).

    A. right root of lung

    B. oblique fissure

    C. horizontal fissure

    D. bronchopulmonary segments

    E. cardiac notch

16. The left lung is divided into two lobes, they are (   ).

    A. lateral lobe

    B. middle lobe

    C. superior lobe

    D. medial lobe

    E. inferior lobe

17. Which ones of the following about lungs are true? (   )

    A. The lungs in fetal can float in water.

    B. The healthy lungs do not contain the air.

    C. The lungs are grey at birth.

    D. The two lungs are separated by mediastinum.

    E. The lungs are situated within the thorax.

18. Which ones of the following are on the anterior border of left lung? (   )

    A. Hilum of left lung

    B. Root of left lung

    C. Cardiac notch of left lung

    D. Lingula of left lung

    E. Cardiac apical incisure

19. Which ones of the following are on the medial surface of right lung? (   )

    A. Lingula of lung

    B. Root of lung

    C. Cardiac notch

    D. Hilum of lung

    E. Cardiac apical incisure

20. The lung possesses two surfaces. They are (   ).

    A. mediastinal surface

    B. lateral surface

    C. costal surface

    D. superior surface

    E. apex surface

21. The pleura is divided into (   ).

    A. parietal pleura

    B. visceral pleura

    C. costal pleura

    D. cupula of pleura

    E. diaphragmatic pleura

22. Which ones of the following belong to the pleural cavity? (   )

    A. Costodiaphragmatic recess

    B. Rectouterine pouch

    C. Rectovesical pouch

    D. Costomediastinal recess

    E. Vesicouterine pouch

23. The mediastinum is divided by the level of the sternal angle into (   ).

    A. posterior mediastinum

    B. superior mediastinum

    C. inferior mediastinum

    D. middle mediastinum

    E. anterior mediastinum

24. The organs located in the posterior mediastinum are (   ).

    A. pericardium

    B. thymus

    C. heart

    D. esophagus

    E. bronchi

25. The organs located in the middle mediastinum are (   ).

    A. esophagus

    B. bronchi

    C. pericardium

    D. heart

    E. vagus

III. Fill the blanks (Fill the most appropriate words in the blanks)

1. The respiratory system includes _____ and _____.

2. _____, _____ and _____ project from the lateral wall of the nasal cavity and subdivide the nasal meatuses.

3. The paranasal sinuses include _____, _____, _____ and _____ four pairs.

4. The sphenoidal sinuses open into _____.

5. _____ is the common channel for both alimentary system and respiratory system.

6. The larynx lies in the neck region in front of _____ vertebrae.

7. The laryngeal cartilages include _____, _____, _____ and _____.

8. The laryngeal vestibule extends from _____ to _____.

9. The infraglottic cavity lies below _____ and extends downward to the lower border of _____.

10. _____ is a sagittal semilunar ridge inside the bifurcation of trachea.

11. The trachea terminates at the level of _____ and divided into _____ and _____.

12. Bronchial tree is composed of _____, _____, _____ and _____.

13. The structures entering and emerging the hilum of lung is called _____.

14. The left lung is divided into _____ and _____ by _____.

15. The right lung is divided into _____, _____ and _____ by _____ and _____.

16. The anterior border of left lung has a deep notch called _____, beneath which is _____.

17. The base of lung is also called _____.

18. The potential space between _____ and _____ is called the pleural cavity.

19. _____ is generally defined as the interval between the right and left pleural sacs.

20. The inferior mediastinum is subdivided into _____, _____ and _____.

IV. Answer questions briefly

1. Please describe the features of trachea.

2. Please describe the features of the right and left principal bronchi.

3. Please describe the position and parts of the lungs.

4. Please describe the parts of pleura.

5. Please describe the parts of mediastinum.

V. Answer questions in detail

1. Please describe the position and opening of the paranasal sinuses.
2. Please describe the shape and parts of laryngeal cavity.
3. Please describe the shape of the lungs.

VI. Problems in life

Why are nose bleeds so common?

Chapter 7   The Urinary System

I . **Single choice (Choose the best answer among the following four choices, and write down the corresponding letter in bracket)**

1. About the shape of the kidney, which is the correct description? (   )

    A. The medial border is convex.

    B. The anterior surface is plane.

    C. It is a pair of chestnut-shaped organs.

    D. The right kidney is broader and shorter than the left.

2. Two or three minor renal calices converge into one (   ).

    A. renal papilla

    B. renal sinus

    C. major renal calyx

    D. renal pelvis

3. Which of the following surrounds the renal papillae? (   )

    A. Minor renal calices

    B. Major renal calices

    C. Renal column

    D. Renal pelvis

4. From the front backward, the order of these structures in the renal pedicle is (   ).

    A. renal artery, renal vein, renal pelvis

    B. renal artery, renal pelvis, renal vein

    C. renal vein, renal artery, renal pelvis

    D. renal pelvis, renal vein, renal artery

5. From superior to inferior, the order of these structures in the renal pedicle is (   ).

    A. renal artery, renal vein, renal pelvis

    B. renal artery, renal pelvis, renal vein

    C. renal vein, renal artery, renal pelvis

    D. renal pelvis, renal vein, renal artery

6. The renal hilum is at the level of (   ) .

    A. fourth thoracic vertebra

    B. first thoracic vertebra

    C. fourth lumbar vertebra

    D. first lumbar vertebra

7. The structure that does **not** pass through the renal hilum is (   ).

   A. renal artery

   B. ureter

   C. renal pelvis

   D. renal vein

8. The structures in the renal pedicle do **not** include (   ) .

   A. renal artery

   B. renal vein

   C. renal pelvis

   D. renal sinus

9. The coverings that is close to the kidney surface is (   ).

   A. fibrous capsule

   B. adipose capsule

   C. renal fascia

   D. visceral peritoneum

10. The left twelfth rib is behind (   ).

    A. the superior part of the posterior surface of the left kidney

    B. the middle part of the posterior surface of the right kidney

    C. the middle part of the posterior surface of the left kidney

    D. the superior part of the posterior surface of the right kidney

11. The right twelfth rib is behind (   ).

    A. the superior part of the posterior surface of the left kidney

    B. the middle part of the posterior surface of the right kidney

    C. the middle part of the posterior surface of the left kidney

    D. the superior part of the posterior surface of the right kidney

12. The structure that transports urine out of the kidney is (   ).

    A. renal papillae

    B. internal urethral orifice

    C. renal pelvis

    D. ureteric orifice

13. There is a vertical slit on medial border of the kidney, it is (   ).

    A. renal hilum

    B. renal pelvis

    C. renal pedicle

    D. renal sinus

14. The superior extremity of the right kidney is at level of (   ).

    A. inferior border of the body of the eleventh thoracic vertebra

    B. superior border of the body of the twelfth thoracic vertebra

    C. inferior border of the body of the second lumbar vertebra

D. superior border of the body of the third lumbar vertebra

15. Which lies immediately beneath the fibrous capsule of kidney? (   )

    A. Renal columns

    B. Renal medulla

    C. Renal cortex

    D. Renal pyramids

16. The renal pyramids belong to (   ).

    A. renal cortex

    B. renal medulla

    C. renal sinus

    D. adipose capsule

17. The structures from renal cortex dipping in between the pyramids are (   ).

    A. renal columns

    B. renal papilla

    C. renal glomeruli

    D. renal medulla

18. Which of the following does the urine formed in the kidney pass through into the calices? (   )

    A. Renal columns

    B. Papillary foramina

    C. Renal hilum

    D. Renal sinus

19. Which of the following does **not** belong to the parts of the ureter? (   )

    A. Abdominal part

    B. Pelvic part

    C. Intramural part

    D. Thorax part

20. The left ureter crosses with (   ).

    A. terminal part of the left common iliac artery anteriorly

    B. terminal part of the left external iliac artery anteriorly

    C. beginning of the left external iliac artery anteriorly

    D. beginning of the left common iliac artery anteriorly

21. The right ureter passes through (   ).

    A. terminal part of the right common iliac artery anteriorly

    B. terminal part of the right external iliac artery anteriorly

    C. beginning of the right external iliac artery anteriorly

    D. beginning of the right common iliac artery anteriorly

22. Which of the following does **not** belong to constrictions of ureter? (   )

    A. At the junction of the ureter and the renal pelvis

B. The part in front of the psoas major

C. At the point where ureter crosses the superior aperture of the lesser pelvis

D. At the intramural part

23. There is a smooth area on the mucosa of internal surface of bladder called (　　).

A. trigone of bladder

B. apex of bladder

C. body of bladder

D. neck of bladder

24. Above the fundus of bladder, which crosses the ureter anteriorly in male? (　　)

A. Spermatic cord

B. Seminal vesicle

C. Ejaculatory duct

D. Ductus deferens

25. The lowest part of urinary bladder is (　　).

A. body of bladder

B. neck of bladder

C. apex of bladder

D. fundus of bladder

26. Which of the following is the landmark to find the ureteric orifices with cystoscope?
(　　)

A. Interureteric ridge

B. Internal urethral orifice

C. Trigone of bladder

D. External urethral orifice

27. Which of the following is **not** behind the fundus of bladder in male? (　　)

A. Seminal vesicles

B. Ampulla of ductus deferens

C. Rectum

D. Urethra

28. In the female, the neck of bladder is attached inferiorly to (　　).

A. urogenital diaphragm

B. rectum

C. pelvic diaphragm

D. uterus

29. In the male, the neck of bladder is attached inferiorly to (　　).

A. pelvic diaphragm

B. urogenital diaphragm

C. prostate gland

D. rectum

30. The largest of the urethral gland in female is (   ).

    A. greater vestibular gland

    B. paraurethral glands

    C. prostate gland

    D. bulbourethral gland

Ⅱ. Double choices(Choose the two best answers among the following choices, and write down the corresponding letters in bracket)

1. The functions of the kidney are (   ).

    A. to excrete the waste products

    B. to reproduce offspring

    C. to supply the body with oxygen

    D. to have endocrine function

    E. to absorb the nutrients

2. The renal region in clinic is between (   ).

    A. lateral border of the psoas major

    B. tenth rib

    C. lateral border of the erector spinae

    D. eleventh rib

    E. twelfth rib

3. On the coronal section of kidney, the renal tissue is divided into (   ).

    A. renal cortex

    B. renal medulla

    C. renal pyramids

    D. renal columns

    E. renal papilla

4. About the renal cortex, which statements are correct? (   ).

    A. It arches over the bases of the minor renal calyx.

    B. It has the renal columns.

    C. It is rich in blood vessels and reddish-brown in color.

    D. It lies beneath the adipose capsule.

    E. It is composed of minor renal calices and major renal calices.

5. Which ones of the following are located in the renal sinus? (   )

    A. Minor renal calices

    B. Renal pyramid

    C. Major renal calices

    D. Renal column

    E. Renal papilla

6. The renal cortex is composed of (   ).

A. renal glomeruli

B. renal pelvis

C. renal pyramids

D. renal papilla

E. renal tubules

7. About the location of kidneys, which two of the following are true? (　　)

A. The left kidney is lower than the right one.

B. The distance between the superior extremities is longer than that between the inferior extremities.

C. It lies on the posterior abdominal wall.

D. It lies on each side of the vertebral column.

E. The inferior extremity of the left kidney is at level of the inferior border of the body of the 11th thoracic vertebra.

8. About the ureter, which descriptions are **wrong**? (　　)

A. It is a pair of muscular tubes.

B. It is divided into two parts: abdominal and pelvic parts.

C. It is to convey the urine from the renal pelvis to the urinary bladder.

D. It has two constrictions.

E. It is 20 – 30 cm in length.

9. The location of abdominal part of ureter is (　　).

A. in front of the psoas major

B. in front of the peritoneum

C. behind the psoas major

D. behind the peritoneum

E. in the mediastinum

10. The uppermost constriction of the ureter is at the junction of (　　).

A. intramural part

B. superior aperture of the lesser pelvis

C. pelvic part

D. renal pelvis

E. ureter

11. Which ones of the following are located behind the fundus of bladder in the female?
(　　)

A. Rectum

B. Upper portion of the vagina

C. Urethra

D. Pubic symphysis

E. Cervix of uterus

12. About the bladder, which statements are correct? (　　)

    A. It is an intraperitoneal organ.

    B. It can produce urine.

    C. It varies in size, shape, position and relations.

    D. Its volume in male is less than in female.

    E. It is a parenchymatous organ.

13. The trigone of bladder is located between (   ).

    A. neck of bladder

    B. ureteric orifices

    C. external urethral orifice

    D. internal urethral orifice

    E. pubic symphysis

14. Which ones of the following do **not** belong to the urinary bladder? (   )

    A. Body of bladder

    B. Head of bladder

    C. Tail of bladder

    D. Neck of bladder

    E. Apex of bladder

15. About the female urethra, which descriptions are correct? (   )

    A. It extends from the bladder to internal urethral orifice.

    B. It perforates the urogenital diaphragm.

    C. Its external orifice is situated behind the vaginal orifice.

    D. It is ventral to the pubic symphysis.

    E. There is the urethrovaginal sphincter.

Ⅲ. Fill the blanks (Fill the most appropriate words in the blanks)

1. _____, _____, _____ and _____ make up the urinary system.

2. The three layers of coverings of kidneys are _____, _____ and _____.

3. Two or three apices of renal pyramids converge in one _____.

4. From the front backward, the order of these structures in the renal pedicle is _____, _____, _____.

5. From superior to inferior, the order of these structures in the renal pedicle is _____, _____, _____.

6. The renal sinus is filled with _____, _____, _____, the branches of renal artery and vein, nerves and adipose tissue.

7. The renal tissue is divided into two portions: _____ and _____.

8. The ureters may be divided into three parts: _____, _____, _____.

9. The trigone of bladder is a smooth triangular area between _____ and _____.

10. The urinary bladder may be divided into four portion: _____, _____, _____ and _____.

Ⅳ. Answer questions briefly

1. Please describe the parts of the ureters.

2. Please describe the constriction of the ureters.

3. Please describe the parts of the urinary bladder.

4. Please describe trigone of bladder.

5. Please describe the feature of the female urethra.

Ⅴ. Answer questions in detail

1. Please describe the shape and location of the kidneys.

2. Please describe the structure of kidney on the coronal section.

Ⅵ. Problems in life

Why does beer stimulate the need to urinate?

Chapter 8   The Reproductive System

Male Reproductive System

I. **Single choice（Choose the best answer among the following four choices, and write down the corresponding letter in bracket）**

　1. Which of the following is **not** the constriction of the male urethra? （　）

　　A. Internal urethral orifice

　　B. External urethral orifice

　　C. Membranous part

　　D. Prostatic part

　2. The male genital ducts which convey the sperm are （　）.

　　A. epididymis and ductus deferens

　　B. ejaculatory duct and ductus deferens

　　C. urethra

　　D. all of above

　3. About the ejaculatory duct, which of the following is true? （　）

　　A. It is a continuation of the ductus deferens.

　　B. It is formed by the union of two ductus deferens.

　　C. It perforates the base of the prostate and enters the prostatic portion of the urethra.

　　D. It opens to the membranous part of the urethra.

　4. Which of the following statements about the testis is **not** true? （　）

　　A. There are two testes, which are housed in the scrotum.

　　B. The testis is covered by the tunica albuginea, which forms the mediastinum testis.

　　C. Each testis is divided into a series of lobules by the septula testis.

　　D. The testis only produces the sperms.

　5. The structures which form the spermatic cord do **not** include （　）.

　　A. ductus deferens

　　B. testicular artery and pampiniform plexus of vein

　　C. nervous plexus and lymphatic system

　　D. epididymis

　6. About the seminal vesicles, which of the following is true? （　）

　　A. They are placed lateral to the urinary bladder.

B. They are placed medial to the ampulla of ductus deferens.

C. They are posterior to the prostate.

D. They are in front of the rectum.

7. About the ejaculatory duct, which one of the following is correct? (　　)

A. It is the beginning of the ductus deferens.

B. It is formed by the union of the end of the ductus deferens and the seminal vesicle duct.

C. It is divided into 2 parts.

D. It opens into the bulb portion of urethra.

8. Male internal reproductive organs include the following structures, **except** (　　).

A. scrotum

B. testis

C. ductus deferens

D. bulbourethral gland

9. Which of the following about ureter is **not** correct? (　　)

A. It is hollow muscular tube.

B. There are three constrictions on each one.

C. It may be divided into two parts such as abdominal and pelvic parts.

D. It is continuous with the renal pelvis at the level of the inferior extremity of the kidney.

10. The second constriction of the ureter is (　　).

A. hilum of the kidney

B. inferior extremity of the kidney

C. the point where ureter crosses with the superior aperture of the lesser pelvis

D. intramural part

11. Which of the statements about the prostate is correct? (　　)

A. Its anterior surface is covered by the peritoneum.

B. Its posterior surface is covered by the peritoneum.

C. It lies below the urinary bladder.

D. It is divided into four lobes.

12. Which of the following statements about the scrotum is **not** true? (　　)

A. It is a pouch of skin and superficial fascia.

B. The superficial fascia contains the smooth muscle fibers to form dartos.

C. The septum of scrotum is composed of skin and dartos.

D. There are two cavities in the scrotum.

13. About the tunica vaginalis of the testis, which statement is **not** correct? (　　)

A. It is made up of the peritoneum.

B. It is divided into parietal and visceral layers.

C. There is serous cavity between the parietal and visceral layers.

      D. The serous cavity communicates with the peritoneal cavity normally.

14. Which of the statement about the penis is correct? (　　)

    A. It has a glans, a body and a root.

    B. It is composed of a cavernous body of penis and a cavernous body of urethra.

    C. The posterior part of the cavernous body of urethra is called the crus penis.

    D. The glans of penis is an enlarged region of the anterior part of the cavernous car-venous body of penis.

15. The testes develop in (　　).

    A. scrotum

    B. abdominal cavity

    C. extraperitoneal space

    D. rectus sheath

16. The organ that secrets androgen is (　　).

    A. thymus

    B. testis

    C. hypophysis

    D. thyroid gland

17. The cremaster muscle comes from (　　).

    A. obliquus externus abdominis and obliquus internus abdominis

    B. obliquus externus abdominis and transversus abdominis

    C. obliquus internus abdominis and transversus abdominis

    D. obliquus externus abdominis

18. The cremaster muscle is innervated by (　　).

    A. genital branch of the genitofemoral nerve

    B. ilioinguinal nerve

    C. T_{12} nerve

    D. femoral nerve

19. The distal (third) stricture of male urethra is at (　　).

    A. internal urethral orifice

    B. membranous part

    C. external urethral orifice

    D. prostatic part

20. All of the following nerves contribute branches to the scrotum, **except** (　　).

    A. lateral femoral cutaneous nerve

    B. pudendal nerve

    C. ilioinguinal nerve

    D. genitofemoral nerve

21. The epididymis is located on the posterior aspect of (　　).

    A. urinary bladder

B. prostate

C. testis

D. ovary

22. The testes are covered by a tough fibrous coat known as the (　　).

A. cremaster fascia

B. tunica albuginea

C. gubernaculum

D. tunica dartos

23. Which of the gland lies below the urinary bladder? (　　)

A. Seminal vesicle

B. Bulbourethral gland

C. Prostate

D. Greater vestibular gland

24. Which part of the ductus deferens can be easy palpated under the skin? (　　)

A. Testicular part

B. Pelvic part

C. Inguinal part

D. Funicular part

25. The penis can be divided into (　　).

A. glans, body and root

B. glans, body and tail

C. glans, neck and body

D. glans, neck and crus

26. Which of the following is the function of the epididymis? (　　)

A. Sperm maturation and storage

B. Produces the bulk of seminal fluid

C. Provides nitric oxide needed for erections

D. Spermatogenesis

27. Spermatogenesis takes place in (　　).

A. prostate

B. penis

C. seminiferous tubules

D. ejaculatory duct

28. Which of the following is the widest and most dilatable portion of the male urethra?
(　　)

A. Navicular fossa

B. Prostatic portion

C. Membranous portion

D. Cavernous portion

29. Which of the following structures opens into the prostatic portion of the male urethra? (   )

A. Ductus deferens

B. Seminal vesicle

C. Ejaculatory duct

D. Bulbourethral gland

30. The mark of the ureteric orifice in clinic is (   ).

A. uvula of bladder

B. trigone of bladder

C. internal urethral orifice

D. interureteric fold

II. Double choices (Choose the two best answers among the following choices, and write down the corresponding letters in bracket)

1. Which structures do **not** belong to the ducts of sperm? (   )

A. Seminal vesical duct

B. Male urethra

C. Ejaculatory duct

D. Ductus deferens

E. Testis

2. Concerning the prostate, which ones of the descriptions are right? (   )

A. Its secretion is the important component of the seminal fluid.

B. It is at the back of the rectum.

C. The urethra passes through it.

D. It is a common gland for male and female.

E. Its base is inferior and against the body of the bladder.

3. Concerning the ductus deferens, which ones of the descriptions are right? (   )

A. Testicular part extends from the tail of epididymis to the superior extremity of testis.

B. Inguinal part extends from the superficial to deep inguinal rings.

C. Pelvic part extends form superior extremity of testis to the superficial inguinal ring.

D. Funicular part crosses the obturator vessels and nerves.

E. Each ductus deferens is divided into 5 parts.

4. Concerning the male urethra, which ones of the descriptions are right? (   )

A. Cavernous part is the widest and most dilatable portion of urethra.

B. Prostatic part transverses the cavernous body of urethra.

C. Membranous part passes through the urogenital diaphragm.

D. It comprises of 3 parts.

E. It comprises of 4 parts.

5. Concerning the prostate, which ones of the following are right? (   )

    A. It lies behind pubic symphysis, between neck of bladder and urogenital dia-phragm.

    B. It contains 5 lobes.

    C. It lies in the deep transverse muscle of perineum.

    D. It opens into bulbar portion of urethra.

    E. It belongs to the external reproductive organs.

6. Concerning the ejaculatory duct, which ones of the descriptions are right? (   )

    A. It secretes part of seminal fluid (60%).

    B. It is formed by union of distal portion of ductus deferens and duct of seminal vesicle.

    C. It passes through the upper part of prostate and opens into the prostatic part of u-rethra.

    D. It contains of 4 parts.

    E. It contains of 3 parts.

7. About the testis, which ones of the descriptions are **wrong**? (   )

    A. It is the gonad in male.

    B. It has two extremities, two surfaces and two borders.

    C. It is suspended in the scrotum by the spermatic cord.

    D. The anterior border connects with the epididymis.

    E. It is the principal storehouse for sperms.

8. Concerning the epididymitis, which ones of the descriptions are right? (   )

    A. It is a thick-walled muscular tube approximately 50 cm in length.

    B. It extends form superior extremity of testis to the superficial inguinal ring.

    C. It is the site of sperm maturation and storage of sperm.

    D. It is located on superior extremity and posterolateral aspect of testis.

    E. It contains of 4 parts.

9. Male internal reproductive organs include the following, **except** (   )

    A. scrotum

    B. penis

    C. epididymitis

    D. ejaculatory duct

    E. prostate

10. The epididymis consists of three parts, **except** (   ).

    A. head

    B. neck

    C. body

    D. tail

    E. apex

III. Fill the blanks (Fill the most appropriate words in the blanks)

1. The male urethra can be divided into three parts, they are _____, _____ and _____.

2. The male urethra has two curvatures, _____ and _____.

3. The ejaculatory duct is formed the union of _____ and _____.

4. The _____ muscle in the spermatic cord can elevate the testes.

5. The accessory glands in male are _____, _____, and _____.

6. The site of sperm maturation and storage is _____.

7. The epididymitis contains the _____, _____ and _____.

8. The ductus deferens is divided into 4 parts: _____, _____, _____, and _____.

9. The prostate contains five lobes, they are _____, _____, _____, _____ and _____.

10. The male urethra has three constrictions, they are _____, _____, _____ and _____.

IV. Answer questions briefly

1. Please describe the internal genital organs of male reproductive system.

2. Please describe the production and storage of sperm and the way to exclude it outside of body.

3. Please describe the contents and coverings of the spermatic cord.

4. Please describe the composition of the ejaculatory duct.

5. Please describe the location, shape and function of prostate.

V. Answer questions in detail

1. Please describe the location and structures of testis.

2. Please describe the course and parts of the ductus deferens.

3. Please describe the characteristics of the male urethra.

VI. Problems in life

During a routine physical examination for a male, why does the physician insert a finger in the superficial inguinal ring under the scrotum and ask the patient to cough?

Female Reproductive System

I. Single choice (Choose the best answer among the following four choices, and write down the corresponding letter in bracket)

1. Concerning the female urethra, which of the following is true? (   )

    A. It is in front of the vagina.

    B. It is in front of the uterus.

    C. It is longer than male urethra.

    D. It lies behind the vaginal vestibule.

2. The ovaries are situated (　　　).

    A. on lateral wall of the lesser pelvis

    B. on posterior wall of the lesser pelvis

    C. in the abdominal cavity

    D. in front of the broad ligament

3. Concerning the ovary, which of the following is true? (　　)

    A. It is covered by anterior layer of broad ligament.

    B. The posterior border has the hilum of ovary.

    C. Its superior extremity has the proper ligament.

    D. Its inferior extremity has the proper ligament.

4. An ovum is usually fertilized in (　　).

    A. infundibulum of uterine tube

    B. ampulla of uterine tube

    C. isthmus of uterine tube

    D. uterine part of uterine tube

5. The longest part of the uterine tube is (　　).

    A. isthmus

    B. infundibulum

    C. ampulla

    D. uterine part

6. Which of the following statements about the uterus is **wrong**? (　　)

    A. The uterus is an organ, in which the fertilized ovum will develop.

    B. It can be divided into three parts: the fundus, body and vaginal part.

    C. The internal cavity is divided into two parts.

    D. The isthmus is a portion between body and cervix.

7. Which of the following statements about the location of the uterus is true? (　　)

    A. Between the urinary bladder and the vagina.

    B. The fundus of the uterus is above the level of the superior circumference of the lesser pelvis.

    C. The inferior end of the cervix is below the ischial spine.

    D. In adult, the position of the uterus is anteflexion and anteversion.

8. The main supports of the uterus are (　　).

    A. muscles of the pelvic floor and neighboring organs

    B. broad ligament and cardinal ligament

    C. round ligament

D. uterosacral ligament

9. Concerning the isthmus of uterus, which of the following is true? (   )

   A. It is the inferior part of the cervix.

   B. It is the narrowest portion of the uterine cavity.

   C. During pregnancy, it is only 1 cm long.

   D. It is the narrowest portion between the body and cervix of the uterus.

10. The function of ovary is (   ).

    A. to produce ova and secrete estrogens

    B. fertilization

    C. storage of sperm

    D. to secrete androgens

11. Which ligament can prevent the uterus from dropping down? (   )

    A. Broad ligament

    B. Round ligament

    C. Cardinal ligament

    D. Uterosacral ligament

12. Concerning the vagina, which of the following is true? (   )

    A. The upper end surrounds the supravaginal portion of the cervix of the uterus.

    B. The posterior fornix is close to the vesicouterine pouch.

    C. The posterior fornix is close to the rectouterine pouch.

    D. The orifice of vagina is in front of the external orifice of urethra.

13. Which of the following lies in the superficial perineal space? (   )

    A. Clitoris

    B. Hymen

    C. Bulbourethral gland

    D. Greater vestibular gland

14. Which of the following is the deepest part of the fornix of vagina? (   )

    A. Anterior fornix

    B. Posterior fornix

    C. Left fornix

    D. Right fornix

15. Concerning the uterus, which of the following is **wrong**? (   )

    A. It is anteverted.

    B. It is anteflexed.

    C. The position of the uterus is fixed.

    D. Interior cavity is divided into two parts.

16. Which part of uterus protrudes into the uppermost of vagina? (   )

    A. Body

    B. Fundus

C. Isthmus

D. Cervix

17. The cervix of the uterus communicates with the vagina via (   ).

A. uterine orifice

B. external orifice

C. abdominal orifice

D. internal orifice

18. Which of the following anchors the ovary laterally to the pelvic wall? (   )

A. Mesovarium

B. Broad ligament of uterus

C. Proper ligament of ovary

D. Suspensory ligament of ovary

19. Fertilization usually occurs in (   ).

A. infundibulum of uterine tube

B. ampulla of uterine tube

C. isthmus of uterine tube

D. uterine part of uterine tube

20. Which of the following anchors the ovary medially to the uterus? (   )

A. Mesovarium

B. Broad ligament of uterus

C. Proper ligament of ovary

D. Suspensory ligament of ovary

21. Supporting structures of ovary is (   ).

A. suspensory ligament of ovary

B. round ligament of uterus

C. cardinal ligament of uterus

D. uterosacral ligament of uterus

22. The internal reproductive organ of the female is (   ).

A. mons pubis

B. lesser lips of pudendum

C. bulb of vestibule

D. vagina

23. About the uterus, which one is **wrong**? (   )

A. It can be divided into four parts, the fundus, body, isthmus and cervix.

B. The isthmus is a slight constriction at the junction between the cervix and body.

C. The lower part of the cervix can insert into the vagina.

D. The cavity of the cervix is called cavity of uterus.

24. About the position of the uterus, which one is **wrong**? (   )

A. Its inferior end is above the ischial spine.

    B. The urinary bladder is in front of it.

    C. The uterine tubes, ovaries, broad ligament are on both sides of it.

    D. It is behind the rectum.

25. Which of the following statements relating to the lesser lips of pudendum is **wrong**?
(   )

    A. They are folds of fat.

    B. They belong to the external reproductive organs.

    C. They are enclosed by the greater lips of pudendum.

    D. They contain sweat glands.

26. The ligament that protects the uterus from prolapsing is (   ).

    A. broad ligament of uterus

    B. suspensory ligament of ovary

    C. round ligament of uterus

    D. cardinal ligament of uterus

27. Vaginal vestibule contains the following structures, **except** (   ).

    A. exteranl orifice of urethra

    B. vaginal orifioo

    C. orifice of the greater vestibular gland

    D. anus

28. Which one is **wrong** about the vagina? (   )

    A. The upper end surrounds the lower part of cervix of uterus.

    B. The anterior wall is longer than the posterior one.

    C. The posterior fornix of vagina is near the rectouterine pouch.

    D. The anterior wall contacts with urinary bladder and urethra.

29. Which of the following extends into the greater lips of pudendum? (   )

    A. Suspensory ligament of ovary

    B. Proper ligament of ovary

    C. Round ligament of uterus

    D. Uterine tube

30. About the uterine tube, which one is **wrong**? (   )

    A. It is situated on the upper margin of the broad ligament of uterus.

    B. Its medial end opens into the cavity of uterus by uterine orifice.

    C. Its lateral end opens into the peritoneal cavity by abdominal orifice.

    D. It can be divided into three part: isthmus, ampulla, and infundibulum.

II . Double choices (Choose the two best answers among the following choices, and write down the corresponding letters in bracket)

1. Concerning the uterus, which ones of the descriptions are right? (   )

    A. It is divided into four portions: fundus, body, isthmus and the cervix.

　　B. It is located anteriorly in the greater pelvis.

　　C. The anteversion is the angle between the body and the cervix.

　　D. The anteflexion is the angle between the uterus and vagina.

　　E. The isthmus is between the body and cervix.

2. About the supports of uterus, which ones of the descriptions are right? (　　)

　　A. Broad ligament extends from the lateral margin of uterus to lateral wall of the pelvis.

　　B. Round ligament maintains the uterus in the anteverted position.

　　C. Cardinal ligament lies at the upper border of broad ligament.

　　D. Uterosacral ligament passes backward from the fundus of uterus.

　　E. Uterosacral ligament can prevent the uterus from dropping down into the vagina.

3. The functions of ovary are (　　).

　　A. to produce ova

　　B. fertilization

　　C. to secrete estrogens

　　D. storage of sperm

　　E. to secrete androgens

4. Concerning the vagina, which ones of the descriptions are right? (　　)

　　A. The upper end surrounds the lower part of cervix of uterus.

　　B. The anterior wall is longer than the posterior one.

　　C. The posterior fornix of vagina is near the rectouterine pouch.

　　D. The anterior wall contacts with rectum.

　　E. The posterior wall contacts with the anterior wall of urinary bladder and urethra.

5. Concerning the ovary, which ones of the descriptions are right? (　　)

　　A. It is situated in the ovary fossa between the common and internal arteries.

　　B. It is a retroperitoneal organ.

　　C. It is connected to the uterus by proper ligament of ovary at its superior extremity.

　　D. It can produce ova and secrete estrogens.

　　E. It is suspended to the pelvic wall by suspensory ligament of ovary.

6. Supporting structures of ovary are (　　).

　　A. suspensory ligament of ovary

　　B. round ligament of uterus

　　C. proper ligament of ovary

　　D. cardinal ligament of uterus

　　E. uterosacral ligament of uterus

7. The ligation and fertilization usually occur in respectively (　　).

　　A. uterine part of uterine tube

　　B. isthmus of uterine tube

　　C. ampulla of uterine tube

　　D. infundibulum of uterine tube

    E. cavity of uterus

8. Supporting structures of uterus are (   ).

    A. suspensory ligament of ovary

    B. round ligament of uterus

    C. proper ligament of ovary

    D. cardinal ligament of uterus

    E. uterine tube

9. Concerning the position of the uterus, which ones of the descriptions are **wrong**?

    (   )

    A. Its inferior end is below the ischial spine.

    B. The urinary bladder is in front of it.

    C. The uterine tubes, ovaries, broad ligament are on both sides of it.

    D. It is behind the rectum.

    E. It lies in the pelvic cavity.

10. Female external genital organs are (   ).

    A. mons pubis

    B. uterus

    C. ovary

    D. vaginal vestibule

    E. uterine tube

III. Fill the blanks (Fill the most appropriate words in the blanks)

1. Ovary lies in the ovarian fossa in the angle between the _____ and _____ iliac vessels on the lateral pelvic wall _____.

2. Supporting structures of ovary are _____ and _____.

3. The uterine tube is divided into _____, _____, _____ and _____.

4. The collective term for the external genitalia of female is _____.

5. The medial and lateral ends of uterine tube are _____ and _____, respectively.

6. The uterus is divided into _____, _____, _____ and _____ four parts.

7. The structure which provides the natural support for the breast is _____.

8. The interior cavity of uterus are _____ and _____.

9. The ligaments of uterus are _____, _____, _____ and _____.

10. The accessory gland of the female is _____.

IV. Answer questions briefly

1. Please describe the internal genital organs of female reproductive system.

2. Please describe the location, shape and ligament of ovary.

3. Please describe the parts of uterine tubes.

4. Please describe the parts of interior cavity of uterus.

5. Please describe the fornix of vagina.

V. Answer questions in detail

1. Please describe the position, shapes, parts and orifices of uterine tubes.

2. Please describe the shape, parts, and cavity of uterus.

3. Please describe the position and fixing structures of uterus.

VI. Problems in life

1. Is it possible for a woman to become pregnant if the man does not ejaculate during sexual intercourse?

2. Have you heard the in vitro fertilization and surrogate motherhood?

3. Can women be allergic to sperm?

Chapter 9 The Peritoneum and the Perineum

I. **Single choice (Choose the best answer among the following four choices, and write down the corresponding letter in bracket)**

1. About the peritoneum, which statement is correct? (   )
   A. The peritoneal cavity is also called abdominal cavity.
   B. The perineum is located only on the inner surface of the abdominal wall and the surface of the abdominal organs.
   C. The peritoneal cavity is closed in men and indirectly communicates with the outside in women.
   D. The peritoneum only can support and fixes organs.

2. About the peritoneal cavity, which statement is correct? (   )
   A. It is enclosed by serosa.
   B. It is enclosed by mucosa.
   C. It is enclosed by the abdominal wall.
   D. The peritoneal cavity is the abdominal cavity.

3. Regarding the peritoneal cavity, which statement is **wrong**? (   )
   A. It is closed in male.
   B. It can communicate with the outside indirectly in female.
   C. The cavity contains a small amount of serum.
   D. It contains visceral organs.

4. About the description of relationship between the peritoneum and organs, which one is correct? (   )
   A. Cecum is an extraperitoneal organ.
   B. Spleen is an intraperitoneal organ.
   C. Liver is an intraperitoneal organ.
   D. Ovary is an intraperitoneal organ.

5. Which one belongs to the intraperitoneal organs? (   )
   A. Stomach
   B. Duodenum
   C. Liver
   D. Ascending colon

6. The intraperitoneal organ is (   ).
   A. cecum and colon
   B. ovary and testis
   C. gallbladder and appendix

　　D. sigmoid colon and rectum

7. The intraperitoneal organ is (　　).

　　A. stomach

　　B. vermiform appendix

　　C. pancreas

　　D. descending colon

8. Which one belongs to the intraperitoneal organs? (　　)

　　A. Transverse colon

　　B. Sigmoid colon

　　C. Urinary bladder

　　D. Kidney

9. Which one belongs to the extraperitoneal organs? (　　)

　　A. Uterus

　　B. Pancreas

　　C. Superior part of rectum

　　D. Urinary bladder

10. Which one does **not** belong to the extraperitoneal organs? (　　)

　　A. Pancreas and descending duodenum

　　B. Kidney and adrenal gland

　　C. Rectum and sigmoid colon

　　D. Seminal vesicle and prostate

11. Which one does **not** belong to the structures formed by peritoneum? (　　)

　　A. Omentum

　　B. Mesentery

　　C. All ligaments

　　D. Peritoneal recess

12. Which one belongs to the lesser omentum? (　　)

　　A. Hepatogastric ligaments

　　B. Gastrocolic ligament

　　C. Gastrosplenic ligament

　　D. Superior duodenum

13. Which of the following descriptions of omental bursa is correct? (　　)

　　A. The omental bursa is part of the abdominal cavity.

　　B. It is not communicating with peritoneal cavity.

　　C. It is located behind the stomach, lesser omentum and gastrocolic ligament.

　　D. The lower wall is formed by the duodenum and pancreas.

14. The intestine that has mesentery is (　　).

　　A. descending colon

　　B. sigmoid colon

C. cecum

D. rectum

15. The intestine **without** mesentery is (   ).

A. jejunum and ileum

B. vermiform appendix

C. transverse and sigmoid colons

D. ascending and descending colons

16. The structure formed by the peritoneum is (   ).

A. broad ligament of uterus

B. round ligament of uterus

C. proper ligament of ovary

D. venous ligament

17. The structure which is **not** formed by the peritoneum is (   ).

A. coronary ligament of liver

B. falciform ligament liver

C. round ligament of liver

D. hepatoduodenal ligament

18. The lowest point of peritoneal cavity in female is (   ).

A. ischiorectal fossa

B. rectovesical pouch

C. rectouterine pouch

D. uterovesical pouch

19. The folds and recesses of the anterior abdominal wall do **not** include (   ).

A. hepatorenal recess

B. supravesical fossa

C. median umbilical fold

D. lateral inguinal fossa

20. The lowest point of peritoneal cavity in supine position is (   ).

A. superior duodenal recess

B. inferior duodenal recess

C. retrocecal recess

D. hepatorenal recess

II. **Double choices** (**Choose the two best answersamong the following choices, and write down the corresponding letters in bracket**)

1. The description of peritoneum, which ones of the following are **wrong**? (   )

A. The peritoneum is only related to abdominal organs.

B. The serosa of the abdominal and pelvic organs is the visceral peritoneum.

C. The hepatogastric ligament connect the porta hepatis to the greater curvature of stomach.

　　D. The hepatoduodenal ligament belongs to the lesser omentum.

　　E. The greater omentum has a fixed effect on jejunum and ileum.

2. The description of peritoneum, which ones of the following are correct? (　　)

　　A. The ability of absorption of lower part of the peritoneum is more than the upper part.

　　B. The peritoneum attached to the inner surface of the abdominal and pelvic walls is the parietal peritoneum.

　　C. The visceral peritoneum is located only on the surface of abdominal organs.

　　D. The space surrounded by the parietal and visceral peritoneum is called the peritoneal cavity.

　　E. The peritoneal cavity is closed in female.

3. The intraperitoneal organs include (　　).

　　A. uterus

　　B. fallopian tube

　　C. ovary

　　D. ureter

　　E. urinary bladder

4. The structures that do **not** belong to peritoneum include (　　).

　　A. round ligament of liver

　　B. hepatogastric ligaments

　　C. hepatoduodenal ligaments

　　D. coronary ligament of liver

　　E. venous ligaments

5. About relationship between colon and peritoneum, which ones of the following are correct? (　　)

　　A. The ascending colon is an intraperitoneal organ.

　　B. The transverse colon is an intraperitoneal organ.

　　C. The descending colon is an extraperitoneal organ.

　　D. The sigmoid colon is an intraperitoneal organ.

　　E. The ascending colon is an extraperitoneal organ.

Ⅲ. Fill the blanks (fill the mostappropriate words in the blanks)

1. Those whose surfaces are completely enclosed by the peritoneum are called ＿＿＿＿.

2. Those whose surfaces are mostly enclosed by the peritoneum are called ＿＿＿＿＿.

3. Those whose surfaces are covered by peritoneum only one side are called ＿＿＿＿.

4. The peritoneal structures connected to the greater and lesser curvatures of stomach are called ＿＿＿＿＿ and ＿＿＿＿＿.

5. The lesser omentum can be divided into ＿＿＿＿＿ and ＿＿＿＿＿.

6. There is _____ , _____ and _____ in the hepatoduodenal ligament.

7. Mesenteric intestines include _____ , _____ , _____ and _____ .

8. Peritoneal pouches anterior and posterior to the uterus are _____ and _____ .

9. Generalized perineum can be divided into two triangles, anterior one is _____ , and posterior one is _____ .

10. In the urogenital diaphragm, urethra passes through in male, _____ and ____ _____ in female.

IV. Answer questions briefly

1. Please describe the concept of peritoneal cavity and its pouches in pelvic cavity.

2. Please describe the major structures formed by the peritoneum.

3. Please describe location and divisions of the lesser omentum.

4. Please describe the ligaments of liver formed by the peritoneum.

5. Please describe the concept of urogenital diaphragm and pelvic diaphragm.

V. Answer questions in detail

1. Please describe the relationship between the peritoneum with abdominal and pelvic organs.

2. Please describe the concept and distinction of perineum.

VI. Problems in life

Have you heard the peritonitis?

Part 3　The Circulatory System

Chapter 10　The General Description and the Heart

Ⅰ. **Single choice（Choose the best answer among the following four choices, and write down the corresponding letter in bracket）**

1. Which organ is regarded as a pump in the blood circulation? （　　）
   A. Heart
   B. Artery
   C. Vein
   D. Capillary

2. The vessels conducting the blood to leave the heart are （　　）.
   A. lymphatic vessels
   B. arteries
   C. veins
   D. capillaries

3. The vessels conducting the blood to come back to the heart are （　　）.
   A. arteries
   B. lymphatic vessels
   C. capillaries
   D. veins

4. The vessels where the substance exchange takes place between blood and tissue fluid are （　　）.
   A. arteries
   B. lymphatic vessels
   C. capillaries
   D. veins

5. Where does the systemic circulation start? （　　）
   A. Left atrium
   B. Left ventricle
   C. Right atrium
   D. Right ventricle

6. Where does the pulmonary circulation start? (   )
   A. Left atrium
   B. Left ventricle
   C. Right atrium
   D. Right ventricle

7. Which structure can be found in the right atrium cavity? (   )
   A. Sulcus terminalis
   B. Crista terminalis
   C. Trabeculae carneae
   D. Papillary muscle

8. Which structure is the unique to the right ventricle? (   )
   A. Valve
   B. Papillary muscle
   C. Tendinous cord
   D. Septomarginal trabecula

9. How many openings are there that conduct the blood into left atrium? (   )
   A. 1
   B. 2
   C. 3
   D. 4

10. Which structure divides the left ventricle into inflow and outflow tracts? (   )
    A. Anterior cusp of the bicuspid valve
    B. Posterior cusp of the bicuspid valve
    C. Annulus of the bicuspid valve
    D. Supraventricular crest

11. Which sulcus separates the atrium from ventricle externally? (   )
    A. Anterior interventricular sulcus
    B. Posterior interventricular sulcus
    C. Coronary sulcus
    D. Supraventricular crest

12. The structure marking the line between the atrium proper and sinus venarum cavarum is (   ).
    A. sulcus terminalis
    B. interatrial sulcus
    C. coronary sulcus
    D. supraventricular crest

13. Which one is correct about cardiac base? (   )
    A. It is facing left, backward and upward.
    B. It is formed mainly by right atrium.

C. It is formed mainly by left ventricle.

D. Large vessels connect to it.

14. Which one is correct about cardiac apex? (   )

A. It is facing right, forward and downward.

B. It is formed by right ventricle.

C. It is behind the left 5th intercostal space.

D. It is at the junction of the anterior and posterior interventricular grooves.

15. The triangle of Koch is located in (   ).

A. left atrium

B. left ventricle

C. right ventricle

D. right atrium

16. Which structure is the pacemaker of the heart? (   )

A. Atrioventricular node

B. Sinoatrial node

C. Purkinje fiber

D. His bundle

17. The valves of heart are formed by (   ).

A. epicardium

B. endocardium

C. myocardium

D. bundle

18. Which one passes through the central fibrous body? (   )

A. Internodal tract

B. Atrioventricular bundle

C. Left bundle branch

D. Purkinje fiber

19. About the fibrous skeleton of heart, which one is correct? (   )

A. It is formed by loose connective tissue.

B. Central fibrous body is also named as left fibrous trigone.

C. Right trigone is smaller than the left.

D. It supplies the attachment for valves of heart.

20. Which valve prevents the blood from returning into left ventricle? (   )

A. Mitral valve

B. Tricuspid valve

C. Aortic valve

D. Pulmonary valve

21. Which structure does **not** belong to the tricuspid complex? (   )

A. Annulus of the tricuspid valve

      B. Tricuspid valve

      C. Tendinous cord

      D. Moderator band

22. Which structure is located at the right side of the interatrial septum? (　　)

      A. Right bundle branch

      B. Fossa ovalis

      C. Septomarginal trabecula

      D. Supraventricular crest

23. Which structure passes through the septomarginal trabecula? (　　)

      A. Internodal tract

      B. Atrioventricular bundle

      C. Left bundle branch

      D. Right bundle branch

24. Coronary arteries originate from (　　).

      A. ascending aorta

      B. aortic arch

      C. aortic vestibule

      D. coronary sinus

25. The artery supplying blood to the anterior part of interventricular septum is (　　).

      A. posterior interventricular branch

      B. anterior interventricular branch

      C. anterior branch of left ventricle

      D. circumflex branch

26. About the posterior interventricular branch, which description is correct? (　　)

      A. It arises from the left coronary artery.

      B. It goes together with the middle cardiac vein.

      C. It supplies blood to the sinoatrial node.

      D. It meets the anterior interventricular branch at the cardiac apex.

27. The right ventricle includes (　　).

      A. fossa ovalis

      B. orifice of superior vena cava

      C. bicuspid valve

      D. tricuspid valve

28. About the chamber of right atrium, which statement is correct? (　　)

      A. It is divided into inflow and outflow tracts.

      B. There are only two openings.

      C. There is fossa ovalis on its medial wall.

      D. There is sulcus terminalis in the chamber of right atrium.

29. The vein companying with the anterior interventricular branch is (　　).
   A. great cardiac vein
   B. middle cardiac vein
   C. small cardiac vein
   D. anterior cardiac vein
30. The transverse cardiac sinus is located (　　).
   A. between the aorta, pulmonary trunk and the anterior wall of left atrium
   B. between the posterior wall of left atrium and the posterior wall of pericardium
   C. at the anterior, inferior part of pericardial cavity
   D. outside of the fibrous pericardium
31. Which structure separates the atrium from ventricle externally? (　　)
   A. Anterior interventricular groove
   B. Posterior interventricular groove
   C. Coronary groove
   D. Interatrial groove
32. The heart is located in (　　).
   A. superior mediastinum
   B. anterior mediastinum
   C. middle mediastinum
   D. posterior mediastinum
33. The inferior border of heart is at the level of (　　).
   A. the 5th thoracic vertebra
   B. the 6th thoracic vertebra
   C. the 7th thoracic vertebra
   D. the 8th thoracic vertebra
34. Which one is the thickest among the free wall of the four chambers of the heart?
   (　　)
   A. Left atrium
   B. Left ventricle
   C. Right atrium
   D. Right ventricle
35. Which one has three entrances among the free wall of the four chambers of the heart? (　　)
   A. Left atrium
   B. Left ventricle
   C. Right atrium
   D. Right ventricle

II. Double choices (Choose the two best answers among the following choices, and write down the corresponding letters in bracket)

1. Which structures belong to the right atrium? (   )
   A. Terminal crest
   B. Fossa ovalis
   C. Aortic valve
   D. Pulmonary valve
   E. Tendinous cord

2. Which branches arise from the left coronary artery? (   )
   A. Anterior interventricular branch
   B. Posterior interventricular branch
   C. Circumflex branch
   D. Branch of atrioventricular node
   E. Branch of the sinoatrial node

3. Which branches arise from the right coronary artery? (   )
   A. Anterior interventricular branch
   B. Posterior interventricular branch
   C. Circumflex branch
   D. Branch of atrioventricular node
   E. Left marginal branch

4. Which structures prevent the blood from returning into atrium? (   )
   A. Aortic valve
   B. Pulmonary valve
   C. Bicuspid valve
   D. Tricuspid valve
   E. The valve of coronary sinus

5. Which vessels supply blood to the interventricular septum? (   )
   A. Circumflex branch
   B. Anterior interventricular branch
   C. Posterior interventricular branch
   D. Posterior branch of left ventricle
   E. Anterior branch of left ventricle

6. Which vessels are located in the anterior interventricular groove? (   )
   A. Circumflex branch
   B. Anterior interventricular branch
   C. Posterior interventricular branch
   D. Great cardiac vein
   E. Middle cardiac vein

7. Which structures can work as a pacemaker for the heart? (   )

A. Internodal tract

B. Atrioventricular node

C. Left bundle branch

D. Right bundle branch

E. Sinoatrial node

8. About the pericardium, which statements are correct? (   )

A. It includes fibrous pericardium and serous pericardium.

B. Fibrous pericardium forms the epicardium.

C. Pericardial cavity is between fibrous pericardium and serous pericardium.

D. Transverse sinus is behind the initial portion of the aorta and pulmonary trunk.

E. Serous pericardium is continuous with the external coats of the great vessels.

9. Which structures belong to the right ventricle? (   )

A. Terminal crest

B. Pectinate muscle

C. Septomarginal trabecula

D. Aortic vestibule

E. Papillary muscle

10. Which structures are located in the right side of the interatrial septum? (   )

A. Supraventricular crest

B. Atrioventricular node

C. Fossa ovalis

D. Right bundle branch

E. Septomarginal trabecula

Ⅲ. **Fill the blanks (Fill the most appropriate words in the blanks)**

1. Circulatory system includes _____ and _____.

2. Cardiovascular system includes _____ circulation and _____ circulation.

3. The vessels of cardiovascular system include _____, _____ and _____.

4. The right atrium is divided into _____ and _____.

5. Ventricle is separated by _____ and _____ externally into right and left parts.

6. In the anterior interventricular groove, _____ branch and _____ vein are located.

7. The tricuspid complex includes _____, _____, _____ and _____.

8. The chamber of right ventricle is divided by _____ into inflow and outflow tracts.

9. The chamber of left ventricle is divided by _____ into inflow and outflow tracts.

10. The arteries distributed in the heart are _____ and _____.

11. The entrances of right atrium are _____ , _____ and _____ .

12. The pericardium includes _____ and _____ .

13. The pericardial cavity is enclosed by _____ and _____ .

14. In the conduction system of heart, _____ is located in the junction between the right atrium and the superior vena cava.

15. In the conduction system of heart, _____ passed through the septomarginal trabecula.

Ⅳ. Answer questions briefly

1. Please describe the formation of the cardiovascular system.
2. Please describe great circulation and lesser circulation.
3. Please describe the conduction system of the heart.
4. Please describe the arteries of the heart.
5. Please describe the veins of the heart.

Ⅴ. Answer questions in detail

1. Please describe the location, external features of the heart.
2. Please describe the chamber of the right atrium.
3. Please describe the chamber of the right ventricle.

Ⅵ. Problems in life

1. During a physical examination, what does a physician tap the chest wall while listening with a stethoscope?
2. What is noninvasive cardiac diagnosis?

Chapter 11   The Arteries

Ⅰ. **Single choice** (**Choose the best answer among the following four choices, and write down the corresponding letter in bracket**)

1. Which artery gives off the coronary artery? (   )
   A. Ascending aorta
   B. Aortic arch
   C. Pulmonary trunk
   D. Thoracic aorta

2. Aortic arch gives off the following branches, **except** (   ).
   A. left common carotid artery
   B. left subclavian artery
   C. brachiocephalic trunk
   D. right common carotid artery

3. Thoracic aorta gives off the following branches, **except** (   ).
   A. posterior intercostal artery
   B. subcostal artery
   C. inferior phrenic artery
   D. esophageal artery

4. Which artery is the visceral branch of the thoracic aorta? (   )
   A. Posterior intercostal artery
   B. Subcostal artery
   C. Superior phrenic artery
   D. Esophageal artery

5. Where does the thoracic aorta start? (   )
   A. At the level of 4th thoracic vertebra
   B. At the level of 6th thoracic vertebra
   C. At the level of 7th thoracic vertebra
   D. At the level of 2nd thoracic vertebra

6. About the carotid sinus, which statement is correct? (   )
   A. It is a chemical receptor.
   B. It is a mechanical receptor.
   C. It is behind of the bifurcation of the common carotid artery.
   D. It is the dilatation of the initial point of the external carotid artery.

7. Which artery gives off the middle meningeal artery? (   )
   A. Facial artery

    B. Maxillary artery

    C. Superficial temporal artery

    D. Occipital artery

8. At the junction of the lower border of the mandible and the anterior border of the masseter, which artery can be felt pulse? (   )

    A. Facial artery

    B. Maxillary artery

    C. Lingual artery

    D. Superior thyroid artery

9. About the subclavian artery, which statement is correct? (   )

    A. Right subclavian artery arises from aortic arch.

    B. It passes through the scalene fissure.

    C. It is continued with the brachial artery.

    D. The superior thyroid artery is one branch of it.

10. The subclavian artery gives off the following branches, **except** (   ).

    A. internal thoracic artery

    B. vertebral artery

    C. thyrocervical trunk

    D. common carotid artery

11. Which muscle is based on for the axillary artery division? (   )

    A. Scalenus anterior

    B. Scalenus medius

    C. Pectoralis major

    D. Pectoralis minor

12. The axillary artery gives off the following branches, **except** (   ).

    A. anterior circumflex humeral artery

    B. posterior circumflex humeral artery

    C. thoracoacromial artery

    D. suprascapular artery

13. The lateral thoracic artery arises from (   ).

    A. subclavian artery

    B. axillary artery

    C. brachial artery

    D. internal thoracic artery

14. Which one is correct about the description of brachial artery? (   )

    A. It is continued with subclavian artery.

    B. It has no other branch at arm.

    C. It divides into ulnar artery and radial artery.

    D. Its pulsation cannot be felt.

15. Which one is the branch directly from the celiac trunk? (   )
    A. Left gastric artery
    B. Right gastric artery
    C. Right gastroepiploic artery
    D. Left gastroepiploic artery
16. Which artery is unpaired? (   )
    A. Renal artery
    B. Testicular artery
    C. Superior mesenteric artery
    D. Middle suprarenal artery
17. Which artery is paired? (   )
    A. Renal artery
    B. Celiac trunk
    C. Superior mesenteric artery
    D. Inferior mesenteric artery
18. The proper hepatic artery gives off (   ).
    A. left gastric artery
    B. right gastric artery
    C. right gastroepiploic artery
    D. left gastroepiploic artery
19. The superior mesenteric artery gives off the following branches, **except** (   ).
    A. right colic artery
    B. middle colic artery
    C. superior pancreaticoduodenal artery
    D. ileocolic artery
20. The inferior mesenteric artery gives off the following branches, **except** (   ).
    A. left colic artery
    B. inferior rectal artery
    C. sigmoid artery
    D. superior rectal artery
21. Which artery is the parietal branch of internal iliac artery? (   )
    A. Lumbar artery
    B. Obturator artery
    C. Umbilical artery
    D. Internal pudendal artery
22. The internal iliac artery gives off the following branches, **except** (   ).
    A. superior gluteal artery
    B. inferior gluteal artery
    C. inferior epigastric artery

D. obturator artery

23. The femoral artery gives off the following branches, **except** (   ).

    A. deep femoral artery

    B. superficial iliac circumflex artery

    C. deep iliac circumflex artery

    D. superficial epigastric artery

24. About the popliteal artery, which statement is correct? (   )

    A. It is continued with femoral artery.

    B. It divides into tibial artery and peroneal artery.

    C. It is superficial to the popliteal vein in the popliteal fossa.

    D. There are little anastomoses formed by its branches.

25. The artery supplying blood to the anterior group of muscles of leg is (   ).

    A. anterior tibial artery

    B. posterior tibial artery

    C. peroneal artery

    D. lateral plantar artery

Ⅱ. **Double choices (Choose the two best answers among the following choices, and write down the corresponding letters in bracket)**

1. Which arteries are connected by arterial ligament? (   )

    A. Left pulmonary artery

    B. Right pulmonary artery

    C. Ascending aorta

    D. Aortic arch

    E. Thoracic aorta

2. Which arteries belong to the visceral branch of the thoracic aorta? (   )

    A. Posterior intercostal artery

    B. Subcostal artery

    C. Superior phrenic artery

    D. Esophageal artery

    E. Bronchial artery

3. Which arteries are the terminal branches of the external carotid artery? (   )

    A. Facial artery

    B. Maxillary artery

    C. Superficial temporal artery

    D. Occipital artery

    E. Lingual artery

4. Which arteries supply blood to the thyroid? (   )

    A. Superior thyroid artery

    B. Middle thyroid artery

    C. Inferior thyroid artery

    D. Anterior thyroid artery

    E. Posterior thyroid artery

5. Which branches of the external carotid artery go backward? (   )

    A. Facial artery

    B. Occipital artery

    C. Lingual artery

    D. Maxillary artery

    E. Posterior auricular artery

6. Which vessels are given off by the common hepatic artery? (   )

    A. Right gastric artery

    B. Right gastroepiploic artery

    C. Proper hepatic artery

    D. Cystic artery

    E. Gastroduodenal artery

7. Superficial palmar arch is formed by (   ).

    A. terminal branch of the ulnar artery

    B. superficial palmar branch of the radial artery

    C. terminal branch of the radial artery

    D. superficial palmar branch of the ulnar artery

    E. deep palmar branch of the ulnar artery

8. Deep palmar arch is formed by (   ).

    A. terminal branch of the ulnar artery

    B. superficial palmar branch of the radial artery

    C. terminal branch of the radial artery

    D. superficial palmar branch of the ulnar artery

    E. deep palmar branch of the ulnar artery

9. The superior mesenteric artery gives off the following branches, **except** (   ).

    A. ileocolic artery

    B. right colic artery

    C. left colic artery

    D. middle colic artery

    E. sigmoid artery

10. Which arteries are unpaired? (   )

    A. Renal artery

    B. Lumbar artery

    C. Median sacral artery

    D. Testicular artery

E. Superior rectal artery

11. Which arteries are paired? (   )

    A. Splenic artery

    B. Lumbar artery

    C. Median sacral artery

    D. Testicular artery

    E. Superior rectal artery

12. Which arteries are the branches of the external iliac artery? (   )

    A. Inferior epigastric artery

    B. Superficial iliac circumflex artery

    C. Deep iliac circumflex artery

    D. External pudendal artery

    E. Superficial epigastric artery

13. Which arteries are the parietal branches of the internal iliac artery? (   )

    A. Inferior epigastric artery

    B. superior gluteal artery

    C. Median sacral artery

    D. Lumbar artery

    E. Inferior gluteal artery

14. About the femoral artery, which statements are correct? (   )

    A. It is continued with the internal iliac artery.

    B. It gives off the deep femoral artery.

    C. It goes together with the femoral vein.

    D. It begins in front of the inguinal ligament.

    E. It becomes tibial artery at the popliteal fossa.

15. About the artery of leg, which statements are correct? (   )

    A. The posterior tibial artery is a continuation of the femoral artery.

    B. The peroneal artery is a branch of the anterior tibial artery.

    C. The peroneal artery supply blood to the anterior group of muscle.

    D. The anterior tibial artery is continued as the dorsal artery of the foot.

    E. The posterior tibial artery descends between the superficial and deep layers of the posterior muscles of leg.

Ⅲ. Fill the blanks (Fill the most appropriate words in the blanks)

1. Aorta can be divided into three parts: _____, _____ and _____.

2. Aortic arch gives off _____, _____ and _____ from its convex aspect.

3. The brachiocephalic trunk divides into _____ and _____.

4. A dilatation at the bifurcation of the common carotid artery, detecting the change of

the blood pressure, is _____.

5. The structure behind the bifurcation of the common carotid artery, detecting the change of the composition of the blood, is _____.

6. The terminal branches of the external carotid artery are _____ and _____.

7. The superficial palmar arch is formed by _____ and _____.

8. The unpaired visceral branches of the abdominal artery are _____, _____ and _____.

9. The paired visceral branches of the abdominal artery are _____, _____ and _____.

10. The arteries distribute in the thyroid are _____ and _____.

11. The superior suprarenal artery arises from _____; the inferior suprarenal artery arises from _____.

12. The left gastric artery arises from _____; the right gastric artery arises from _____.

13. The left gastroepiploic artery arises from _____; the right gastroepiploic artery arises from _____.

14. The branches of celiac trunk are _____, _____ and _____.

15. The posterior tibial artery passes behind _____ into planta.

IV. Answer questions briefly

1. Please describe the main branches of the axillary artery.

2. Please describe the location and formation of the superficial palmar arch.

3. Please describe the arteries of the suprarenal gland.

V. Answer questions in detail

1. Please describe the arteries of the stomach.

2. Please describe the course and division of the aorta.

VI. Problems in life

Since blood is already within large arteries and veins, why do these vessels need their own blood supply?

Chapter 12　The Veins

I. **Single choice (Choose the best answer among the following four choices, and write down the corresponding letter in bracket)**

1. About the characteristic of veins, which statement is correct? (　　)
   A. It is as same as the artery in number.
   B. It is smaller than the companying artery.
   C. The venous valve in limb is less than trunk.
   D. There are rich anastomoses among veins.

2. About the systemic vein, which statement is correct? (　　)
   A. It is divided into superficial and deep groups.
   B. The superficial vein goes together with the artery.
   C. The deep veins are commonly used to transfuse, puncture, catheterize and get blood.
   D. There are no anastomoses between superficial veins and deep veins.

3. How many pulmonary veins are there in our body? (　　)
   A. 2
   B. 3
   C. 4
   D. 6

4. The pulmonary veins enter into (　　).
   A. left atrium
   B. right atrium
   C. left ventricle
   D. right ventricle

5. About the facial vein, which statement is correct? (　　)
   A. It originates from the angular vein.
   B. It goes downwards in front of the facial artery at face.
   C. There are rich valves in facial vein.
   D. It ends into the external jugular vein.

6. Which vein is formed by a confluence of the veins in the pterygoid venous plexus? (　　)
   A. Superficial temporal vein
   B. Maxillary vein
   C. Retromandibular vein
   D. Facial vein

7. About superior vena cava, which statement is correct? (   )

   A. It is formed by the left and right internal jugular veins.

   B. It begins behind the lower border of the first left costal cartilage.

   C. It receives the azygos vein before entering into the right atrium.

   D. It ends in the right atrium at the lower border of the third sternocostal joint.

8. About the external jugular vein, which statement is correct? (   )

   A. It is the smallest superficial vein in the neck.

   B. It is formed by the union of the posterior division of the retromandibular vein with the posterior auricular vein.

   C. It ends in the internal jugular vein.

   D. The vein of thyroid is collected by it.

9. Which vein belongs to the deep vein? (   )

   A. Cephalic vein

   B. Basilic vein

   C. Median cubital vein

   D. Radial vein

10. Which vein is usually selected for blood sampling? (   )

    A. Cephalic vein

    B. Basilic vein

    C. Median cubital vein

    D. Dorsal venous rete of hand

11. Which vein is usually selected for intravenous drip? (   )

    A. Cephalic vein

    B. Basilic vein

    C. Median cubital vein

    D. Dorsal venous rete of hand

12. Which vein is the continuation of the right ascending lumbar vein? (   )

    A. Azygos vein

    B. Hemiazygos vein

    C. Accessory hemiazygos vein

    D. Internal thoracic vein

13. Which vein is the continuation of the left ascending lumbar vein? (   )

    A. Azygos vein

    B. Hemiazygos vein

    C. Accessory hemiazygos vein

    D. Internal thoracic vein

14. Which one is correct about the inferior vena cava? (   )

    A. It is smaller than superior vena cava.

    B. It passes through the diaphragm at level of the 10th thoracic vertebra.

    C. It is formed by the junction of the two common iliac vein at the anterior of the 4th lumbar vertebra.

    D. It receives blood from all structures below the diaphragm.

15. Which vein is the parietal tributary of the internal iliac vein? (　　)

    A. Superior rectal vein

    B. Inferior rectal vein

    C. Internal pudendal vein

    D. Superior gluteal vein

16. The following veins are superficial vein in the lower limb, **except** (　　).

    A. great saphenous vein

    B. small saphenous vein

    C. dorsal venous arch of the foot

    D. peroneal vein

17. Which vein runs behind the lateral malleolus? (　　)

    A. Great saphenous vein

    B. Small saphenous vein

    C. Dorsal venous arch of the foot

    D. Peroneal vein

18. The following veins are visceral tributaries of the inferior vena cava, **except** (　　).

    A. lumbar vein

    B. testicular vein

    C. renal vein

    D. right suprarenal vein

19. Which vein is unpaired? (　　)

    A. renal vein

    B. suprarenal vein

    C. superior mesenteric vein

    D. testicular vein

20. Which vein ends in the inferior vena cava directly? (　　)

    A. left suprarenal vein

    B. right suprarenal vein

    C. left testicular vein

    D. hepatic portal vein

21. How many hepatic veins are there generally? (　　)

    A. 1

    B. 2

    C. 3

    D. 4

22. These veins are collected by hepatic portal vein, **except** (　　).

    A. superior mesenteric vein

    B. inferior mesenteric vein

    C. cystic vein

    D. inferior rectal vein

23. The hepatic portal vein is formed behind (   ).

    A. head of pancreas

    B. neck of pancreas

    C. body of pancreas

    D. tail of pancreas

24. About the hepatic portal vein, which statement is correct? (   )

    A. It is formed by the union of the superior and inferior mesenteric veins.

    B. It enters into the liver at the second hepatic porta.

    C. It collects blood from unpaired organs (except the liver) in the abdominal cavity and the rectum in the pelvic cavity.

    D. There are no anastomoses between it and the superior vena cava.

25. Which vein could become large at the situation of the cirrhosis of liver? (   )

    A. Hepatic vein

    B. Inferior vena cava

    C. Hepatic portal vein

    D. Renal vein

Ⅱ. **Double choices (Choose the two best answers among the following choices, and write down the corresponding letters in bracket)**

1. Which ones are the special vein in structure? (   )

    A. Superficial vein

    B. Deep vein

    C. Sinus of dura mater

    D. Portal vein

    E. Diploic vein

2. Retromandibular vein is formed by the union of (   ).

    A. facial vein

    B. maxillary vein

    C. superior thyroid vein

    D. superficial temporal vein

    E. mandibular vein

3. Which veins are the deep vein? (   )

    A. Facial vein

    B. Internal jugular vein

    C. External jugular vein

    D. Cephalic vein

    E. Basilic vein

4. Which veins end into the left renal vein? (　　)

    A. Left suprarenal vein

    B. Left lumbar vein

    C. Left inferior phrenic vein

    D. Superior mesenteric vein

    E. Left testicular vein

5. Hepatic portal vein is formed by the union of (　　).

    A. superior mesenteric vein

    B. inferior mesenteric vein

    C. splenic vein

    D. left gastric vein

    E. right gastric vein

6. Venous angle is formed by (　　).

    A. internal jugular vein

    B. external jugular vein

    C. facial vein

    D. subclavian vein

    E. brachiocephalic vein

7. The blood from the left posterior intercostal veins is collected by (　　).

    A. azygos vein

    B. right lumbar vein

    C. hemiazygos vein

    D. accessory hemiazygos vein

    E. right internal thoracic vein

8. There are rich valves in the following veins, **except** (　　).

    A. great saphenous vein

    B. small saphenous vein

    C. facial vein

    D. cephalic vein

    E. hepatic portal vein

9. Which veins enter into the internal iliac vein? (　　)

    A. Superior rectal vein

    B. Inferior rectal vein

    C. Internal pudendal vein

    D. External pudendal vein

    E. Superficial iliac circumflex vein

10. Which anastomoses are formed between hepatic portal vein and the superior vena ca-

va? (   )

A. Esophageal venous plexus

B. Rectal venous plexus

C. Periumbilical venous plexus

D. Pterygoid venous plexus

E. Uterus venous plexus

III. Fill the blanks (Fill the most appropriate words in the blanks)

1. The main superficial vein in the neck is _____.

2. The superficial veins in the upper limb are _____, _____ and _____.

3. The tributaries of the great saphenous vein are _____, _____, _____, _____ and _____.

4. The special veins in body are _____ and _____.

5. The right suprarenal vein enters into _____; the left suprarenal vein enters into _____.

6. The small saphenous vein enters into _____.

7. The median cubital vein makes a connection between _____ and _____.

8. The right testicular vein enters into _____; the left testicular vein enters into _____.

9. The inferior vena cava ascends at the right of _____, then passes _____ of the liver in abdominal cavity.

10. The main tributaries of external jugular vein are _____, _____ and _____.

IV. Answer questions briefly

1. Please describe the characteristics of the veins.

2. Where is the dangerous area? What is the reason?

3. Please describe the course of the inferior vena cava.

V. Answer questions in detail

1. Please describe the course, tributaries of the great saphenous vein.

2. Please describe the tributaries and anastomoses of the hepatic portal vein.

VI. Problems in life

Why do your nose and cheeks turn red on a cold day?

Chapter 13   The Lymphatic System

Ⅰ. **Single choice（Choose the best answer among the following four choices, and write down the corresponding letter in bracket）**

1. About the characteristics of lymphatic system, which statement is correct? (　　)

    A. The cardiovascular system is an accessory system of lymphatic system.

    B. Most tissue fluid is taken up by the lymphatic capillaries.

    C. The fluid in the lymphatic vessels is termed lymph.

    D. The function of the lymphatic system is only to take part in the immune responses.

2. About the lymph conducting vessels, which statement is correct? (　　)

    A. Lymphatic capillaries begin as dilated blind ends.

    B. Lymphatic vessels have no valves.

    C. There are 8 lymphatic trunks in human body.

    D. The thoracic duct conveys 1/4 of the lymph back to the blood.

3. How many lymphatic trunks are there in body? (　　)

    A. 6

    B. 7

    C. 8

    D. 9

4. The thoracic duct enters into (　　).

    A. left venous angle

    B. right venous angle

    C. left brachiocephalic vein

    D. right brachiocephalic vein

5. The right lymphatic duct enters into (　　).

    A. right internal jugular vein

    B. right venous angle

    C. right atrium

    D. right brachiocephalic vein

6. Which one is **not** a lymphoid organ? (　　)

    A. Lymph node

    B. Spleen

    C. Thymus

    D. Thyroid

7. Lymphatic capillaries join with each other and form (　　).

  A. lymph node

  B. lymphatic vessel

  C. lymphatic trunk

  D. lymphatic duct

8. Lymphatic trunks are received by (　　).

  A. lymph node

  B. lymphatic vessel

  C. vein

  D. lymphatic duct

9. The cisterna chyli lies in front of the (　　).

  A. first lumbar vertebra

  B. second lumbar vertebra

  C. third lumbar vertebra

  D. twelfth thoracic vertebra

10. The ratio of the lymph collected by thoracic duct is (　　).

  A. 1/4

  B. 1/2

  C. 3/4

  D. 1

11. Which node belongs to the lymph nodes of neck? (　　)

  A. Occipital lymph node

  B. Submandibular lymph node

  C. Submental lymph node

  D. Virchow's lymph node

12. How many groups of lymph node are there in axilla? (　　)

  A. 3

  B. 4

  C. 5

  D. 6

13. Which group of lymph nodes receives the lymph from the lower part of the abdominal wall? (　　)

  A. The upper group of the superficial inguinal lymph nodes

  B. The lower group of the superficial inguinal lymph nodes

  C. The deep group of the inguinal lymph nodes

  D. The superficial group of the external iliac lymph nodes

14. The largest lymphoid organ is (　　).

  A. lymph node

  B. thyroid

  C. thymus

D. spleen

15. The spleen is located in the (   ).

   A. left hypochondriac region of the abdomen

   B. right hypochondriac region of the abdomen

   C. epigastric region of the abdomen

   D. hypogastric region of the abdomen

16. The long axis of spleen corresponds to the (   ).

   A. 8th rib

   B. 9th rib

   C. 10th rib

   D. 11th rib

17. The splenic notches are located at/on (   ).

   A. inferior border

   B. superior border

   C. diaphragmatic surface

   D. visceral surface

10. The hilum of spleen is located at/on (   )

   A. inferior border

   B. superior border

   C. diaphragmatic surface

   D. visceral surface

19. The T lymphocytes mature in (   ).

   A. spleen

   B. thymus

   C. thyroid

   D. tonsil

20. The thoracic duct passes into thoracic cavity through (   ).

   A. aortic hiatus of diaphragm

   B. esophageal hiatus of diaphragm

   C. vena cava foramen of diaphragm

   D. right diaphragmatic crus

II. Double choices (Choose the two best answers among the following choices, and write down the corresponding letters in bracket)

1. Which organs are **not** the lymphoid organ? (   )

   A. Liver

   B. Spleen

   C. Lymph node

   D. Thymus

E. Thyroid

2. The thoracic duct does **not** receive (　　).

   A. right jugular trunk

   B. left jugular trunk

   C. right subclavian trunk

   D. left subclavian trunk

   E. intestinal trunk

3. Which trunks enter into the right lymphatic duct? (　　)

   A. Right lumbar trunk

   B. Right jugular trunk

   C. Right intestinal trunk

   D. Right subclavian trunk

   E. Cisterna chyli

4. The superficial inguinal lymph nodes can be divided into (　　).

   A. upper group

   B. lower group

   C. lateral group

   D. posterior group

   E. deep group

5. The efferent lymphatic vessels of the superior part of breast drain into (　　).

   A. apical lymph nodes

   B. subscapular lymph nodes

   C. parasternal lymph nodes

   D. pectoral lymph nodes

   E. supraclavicular lymph nodes

6. Which nodes are along with the external jugular vein or internal jugular vein? (　　)

   A. Superficial lateral cervical lymph nodes

   B. Deep lateral cervical lymph nodes

   C. Superficial anterior cervical lymph nodes

   D. Deep anterior cervical lymph nodes

   E. Carotid lymph nodes

7. Which lymphatic trunks are located in thoracic cavity? (　　)

   A. Thoracic trunk

   B. Left subclavian trunk

   C. Right subclavian trunk

   D. Left bronchomediastinal trunk

   E. Right bronchomediastinal trunk

8. The lymph vessels from the fundus and the superior part of the uterine body drain into (　　).

A. external iliac lymph nodes

B. superficial inguinal lymph nodes

C. deep inguinal lymph nodes

D. lumbar lymph nodes

E. internal iliac lymph nodes

9. The superficial inguinal lymph nodes do **not** receive the lymph from (   ).

A. lower part of anterolateral wall of abdomen

B. superficial lymphatic vessels from lateral margin of foot

C. gluteal region

D. fundus of uterine

E. superficial lymphatic vessels from the posterolateral part of leg

10. Which lymph nodes are along with the axillary vein? (   )

A. Pectoral lymph node

B. Lateral lymph node

C. Subscapular lymph node

D. Central lymph node

D. Apical lymph node

III. Fill the blanks (Fill the most appropriate words in the blanks)

1. The lymphatic system consists of _____ , _____ and _____ .

2. The lymphoid tissues include _____ and _____ .

3. The lymphatic trunks collected by right lymphatic duct are _____ , _____ and _____ .

4. The cisterna chyli is formed by _____ , _____ and _____ .

5. The unpaired lymphatic trunk is _____ .

6. The thoracic duct ends into _____ .

7. The lymphoid organ exerting erythrocyte storage is _____ .

8. Lymph conducting vessels include _____ , _____ , _____ and _____ .

9. The efferent lymphatic vessels leaves the lymph node at _____ .

10. The lymph node receiving the afferents from the ulnar halves of the hand and fore-arm is _____ .

IV. Answer questions briefly

1. Please describe the formation of the lymphatic system.

2. Please describe the number and the name of the lymphatic trunk.

3. Please describe the external feature of the lymph nodes.

4. Please describe the groups of the axillary lymph nodes.

V. Answer questions in detail

1. Please describe the course and the drainage area of the thoracic duct.

2. Please describe the lymphatic drainage of the mammary gland.

Part 4 The Sensory System

Chapter 14 The Visual Organs

Ⅰ. **Single choice（Choose the best answer among the following four choices, and write down the corresponding letter in bracket）**

1. About the ocular axis, which of the following is right? （   ）
   A. It is the line joining the two poles of the eyeball.
   B. It is the line joining the anterior pole and the center of the pupil.
   C. It is the line joining the anterior pole and the fovea centralis of the retina
   D. It is the line joining the center of the pupil and the fovea centralis of the retina.

2. About the optic axis, which of the following is right? （   ）
   A. It is the line joining the two poles of the eyeball.
   B. It is the line joining the anterior pole and the fovea centralis of the retina.
   C. It is the line joining the posterior pole and the fovea centralis of the retina.
   D. It is the line joining the center of the pupil and the fovea centralis of the retina.

3. The anterior one-sixth potion of the eyeball fibrous tunic is （   ）.
   A. retina
   B. cornea
   C. ciliary body
   D. sclera

4. Which of the following structures is a **non-vascular** one? （   ）
   A. Ciliary body
   B. Cornea
   C. Retina
   D. Iris

5. Which of the following structures has the function of controlling the amount of the light entering the eyeball? （   ）
   A. Sclera
   B. Iris
   C. Ciliary body
   D. Retina

6. Which of the following structures does **not** contain pigment cells? (   )

   A. Cornea

   B. Retina

   C. Ciliary body

   D. Iris

7. Aqueous humor is secreted by (   ).

   A. iris

   B. retina

   C. ciliary body

   D. sclera

8. Which of the following muscles can constrict the pupil? (   )

   A. Dilator pupillae

   B. Ciliary zonule

   C. Sphincter pupillae

   D. Ciliary muscle

9. Which of the following structures is attached to the lens? (   )

   A. Dilator pupillae

   B. Ciliary zonule

   C. Sphincter pupillae

   D. Ciliary muscle

10. The chamber of the eyeball is divided into anterior and posterior chambers by

    (   ).

    A. retina

    B. cornea

    C. ciliary body

    D. iris

11. Which structure is responsible for the nutrition of the outer layer of the retina?

    (   )

    A. Sclera

    B. Iris

    C. Ciliary body

    D. Choroid

12. Which structure is responsible for the support of the retina? (   )

    A. Iris

    B. Choroid

    C. Vitreous body

    D. Sclera

13. Which of the following structures is lacking vessels and nerves? (   )

    A. Choroid

B. Lens

C. Ciliary body

D. Sclera

14. The first order neuron of the retina is (   ).

A. rod cell

B. cone cell

C. bipolar cell

D. ganglion cell

15. The second order neuron of the retina is (   ).

A. ganglion cell

B. cone cell

C. bipolar cell

D. rod cell

16. The area with the highest visual acuity is (   ).

A. optic disc

B. fovea centralis

C. iridial part

D. ciliary part

17. The "blind spot" refers to (   ).

A. optic disc

B. fovea centralis

C. iridial part

D. ciliary part

18. Which of the following structures is related to the occurrence of cataract? (   )

A. Optic disc

B. Fovea centralis

C. Lens

D. Vitreous body

19. Which of the following structures is related to the occurrence of retinodialysis?
    (   )

A. Optic disc

B. Fovea centralis

C. Lens

D. Vitreous body

20. Which of the following areas is insensitive to light? (   )

A. Optic disc

B. Fovea centralis

C. Macula lutea

D. Optic part of the retina

21. Which of the following structures belongs to the wall of eyeball? (   )

    A. Aqueous humor

    B. Choroid

    C. Vitreous body

    D. Superior obliquus

22. Which of the following structures belongs to the accessory organs of eye? (   )

    A. Aqueous humor

    B. Choroid

    C. Vitreous body

    D. Lacrimal apparatus

23. The eyelid includes the following structures **except** (   ).

    A. skin

    B. subcutaneous areolar tissue

    C. orbicularis oculi

    D. superior obliquus

24. Which side of optic disc is macula lutea located to? (   )

    A. Nasal

    B. Temporal

    C. Caudal

    D. Rostral

25. The following muscles belong to extraocular muscles **except** (   ).

    A. medial rectus

    B. lateral rectus

    C. orbicularis oculi

    D. superior obliquus

26. Which of the following muscles is responsible for the adjustment of diopter of lens?
    (   )

    A. Medial rectus

    B. Ciliary muscle

    C. Orbicularis oculi

    D. Superior obliquus

27. Which of the following cells take part in the formation of optic nerve? (   )

    A. Ganglion cell

    B. Cone cell

    C. Bipolar cell

    D. Rod cell

28. Which of the following structures is responsible for the nutrition of cornea? (   )

    A. Aqueous humor

    B. Choroid

    C. Vitreous body

    D. Lacrimal apparatus

29. About the lens, which one is **incorrect**? (　　)

    A. It is located between the iris and vitreous body.

    B. It is colorless, transparent and without innervations.

    C. Its diopter changes with the distance.

    D. It is an inelastic structure.

30. The exteroceptors are located in (　　).

    A. heart

    B. joint

    C. skin

    D. muscle

Ⅱ. Double choices (Choose the two best answers among the following choices, and write down the corresponding letters in bracket)

1. The fibrous tunic of the eyeball consists of (　　).

    A. retina

    B. cornea

    C. ciliary body

    D. sclera

    E. iris

2. The vascular tunic of the eyeball consists of the following structures, **except** (　　).

    A. choroid

    B. cornea

    C. ciliary body

    D. sclera

    E. iris

3. The structures which contain pigment cells include (　　).

    A. sclera

    B. cornea

    C. ciliary body

    D. retina

    E. aqueous humor

4. Which ones of the following structures are colorless? (　　)

    A. Retina

    B. Cornea

    C. Ciliary body

    D. Iris

    E. Aqueous humor

5. Which ones of the following structures are transparent? (   )

   A. Retina

   B. Lens

   C. Ciliary body

   D. Iris

   E. Vitreous body

6. The neurons of the retina include (   ).

   A. ganglion cell

   B. cone cell

   C. bipolar cell

   D. rod cell

   E. pigment cell

7. The photoreceptors of the retina include (   ).

   A. ganglion cell

   B. cone cell

   C. bipolar cell

   D. rod cell

   E. pigment cell

8. The exteroceptors are located in (   ).

   A. heart

   B. joint

   C. skin

   D. muscle

   E. nasal and oral mucous membrane

9. Which ones of the following structures belong to the contents of the eyeball? (   )

   A. Retina

   B. Lens

   C. Ciliary body

   D. Iris

   E. Aqueous humor

10. Which ones of the following structures are with refractive effect? (   )

    A. Retina

    B. Cornea

    C. Ciliary body

    D. Iris

    E. Aqueous humor

11. Which ones of the following muscles are controlled by oculomotor nerve? (   )

    A. Medial rectus

    B. Lateral rectus

  C. Orbicularis oculi

  D. Superior obliquus

  E. Superior rectus

12. About the lens, which ones are **incorrect**? ( )

  A. It is located between the iris and vitreous body.

  B. It is colorless and transparent.

  C. Its diopter changes with the distance.

  D. It is an inelastic structure.

  E. It is abundant in nerve innervations.

13. About the cornea, which ones are **incorrect**? ( )

  A. It is the anterior portion of fibrous tunic.

  B. It is colorless and transparent.

  C. It has refractive effect.

  D. It has pigment cells.

  E. It is abundant in blood supply.

14. About the retina, which ones are **incorrect**? ( )

  A. It is the anterior portion of fibrous tunic.

  B. It is colorless and transparent.

  C. It has blind spot.

  D. It has pigment cells.

  E. It has macula lutea.

15. The blind part of the retina includes ( ).

  A. iridial part

  B. macula lutea

  C. blind spot

  D. ciliary part

  E. optic part

Ⅲ. Fill the blanks (Fill the most appropriate words in the blanks)

1. The three tunics of the eyeball are _____, _____ and _____.

2. The fibrous tunic of the eyeball consists of _____ and _____.

3. The vascular tunic of the eyeball consists of _____, _____ and _____.

4. Aqueous humor is secreted by _____.

5. The contents of eyeball include _____, _____ and _____.

6. From the back forward, retina can be divided into three parts, they are _____, _____ and _____.

7. The blind part of retina include _____ and _____.

8. The neurons of the retina include _____ and _____.

9. About the eyeball, the structures which are with refractive effect include _____,

_____ , _____ and _____ .

10. The aqueous humor fills _____ .

11. The blind spot is located at _____ .

12. The site with highest visual acuity is _____ .

13. The part of the fibrous tunic which is with refractive effect is _____ .

14. Pupil is located in the centre of _____ .

15. The extraocular muscles include _____ , _____ , _____ , _____ , _____ and _____ .

IV. Answer questions briefly

1. Please briefly describe those structures of the eyeball that with refractive effect and their location.

2. Please briefly describe the subdivisions of the retina and the location of the macula lutea and optic disc.

3. Please briefly describe the subdivision and the function of the vascular tunic.

4. Please describe the layers of the eyelid.

5. Please describe the extraocular muscles.

V. Answer questions in detail

1. Please describe the extraocular muscle and their nerve supply.

2. Please describe the three tunics of the eyeball and their subdivisions.

3. Please describe the contents of the eyeball and their location and function.

VI. Problems in life

1. What causes "bloodshot eyes"?

2. Why do we sometimes see "spots" in front of our eyes?

3. Why do most newborn babies have blue eyes?

Chapter 15　The Vestibulocochlear Organs

Ⅰ. **Single choice（Choose the best answer among the following four choices, and write down the corresponding letter in bracket）**

1. About the auricle, which of the following is **false**? （　　）

    A. It projects from the side of the head.

    B. It has bony framework.

    C. It is composed of a thin plate of elastic fibrocartilage and covered by skin.

    D. The auricular lobule is composed of fibrous and adipose tissue.

2. About the external acoustic meatus, which of the following is **false**? （　　）

    A. It extends from the external acoustic pore to the tympanic membrane.

    B. It is about 2.1 – 2.5 cm in length.

    C. Its posterosuperior wall is longer than anteroinferior wall.

    D. It comprises cartilaginous part and bony part.

3. About the external acoustic meatus, which of the following is true? （　　）

    A. It is covered by mucous membrane.

    B. There is no sebaceous gland in the subcutaneous tissue of this meatus.

    C. Its lateral 1/3 is termed cartilaginous part.

    D. Its posterosuperior wall is longer than anteroinferior wall.

4. About thetympanic membrane, which of the following is **false**? （　　）

    A. It is oval in appearance.

    B. It separates the middle ear from the external acoustic meatus.

    C. It forms an angle of 45 degrees with the floor of the meatus.

    D. Its lateral surface is covered by mucous membrane.

5. About the tympanic membrane, which of the following is correct? （　　）

    A. It is rectangle in appearance.

    B. It separates the middle ear from the external acoustic meatus.

    C. It forms an angle of 45 degrees with the roof of the meatus.

    D. It is composed of two layers.

6. Which of the following descriptions about the location of the cone of light is right?
    （　　）

    A. It is anteroinferior to the umbo.

    B. It is posterosuperior to the umbo.

    C. It is lateral to the umbo.

    D. It is medial to the umbo.

7. Which of the following statements about the tympanic membrane is right? （　　）

A. The umbo is located on the margin of the membrane.

B. The flaccid part is devoid of skin.

C. Its mucous membrane is continuous with that of the middle ear.

D. The flaccid part is thicker than the tense part.

8. Which of the following is **not** the layer of tympanic membrane? (   )

A. Cuticular layer

B. Mucous layer

C. Fibrous layer

D. Muscular layer

9. About the tympanic membrane, which of the following is **not** true? (   )

A. Cuticular layer is the outer layer.

B. Mucous layer is the inner layer.

C. Fibrous layer is the intermediate layer.

D. Muscular layer is the inner layer.

10. About the tympanic cavity, which of the following is **false**? (   )

A. It is an irregular fluid-filled space.

B. It is located inside the temporal bone.

C. It lies between the tympanic membrane and the lateral wall of the inner ear.

D. There are auditory ossicles inside the tympanic cavity.

11. About the tympanic cavity, which of the following is true? (   )

A. It is an irregular fluid-filled space.

B. It is located inside the occipital bone.

C. It lies between the tympanic membrane and the lateral wall of the inner ear.

D. There are two auditory ossicles inside the tympanic cavity.

12. The lateral wall of the tympanic cavity is also known as (   ).

A. membranous wall

B. jugular wall

C. mastoid wall

D. carotid wall

13. Which of the following structures belongs to the posterior wall of the tympanic cavity? (   )

A. Pyramidal eminence

B. Tympanic membrane

C. Second tympanic membrane

D. Round window

14. Which of the following structures belongs to the medial wall of the tympanic cavity? (   )

A. Pyramidal eminence

B. Fenestra vestibuli

C. Tympanic membrane

D. Opening of the mastoid antrum

15. The fenestra cochlea is closed by (   ).

A. tympanic membrane

B. second tympanic membrane

C. base of stapes and annular ligament

D. spiral membrane

16. About the auditory tube, which one is **incorrect**? (   )

A. It is a channel through which the tympanic cavity communicates with nasopharynx.

B. Its bony part is about two-thirds of its total length.

C. It is approximately 3.5 – 4 cm long.

D. In childhood, the auditory tube is relatively shorter than that in adult.

17. About the inner ear, which one is **incorrect**? (   )

A. It lies in the petrous portion of the temporal bone.

B. It consists of two parts: the bony labyrinth and membranous labyrinth.

C. The membranous labyrinth is composed of a series of membranous sacs and ducts.

D. The membranous labyrinth is filled with perilymph

18. Which of the following statements about the vestibule is **not** correct? (   )

A. The vestibule is the central part of the bony labyrinth.

B. The fenestra vestibuli and fenestra cochlea are located on the lateral wall of the vestibule.

C. On the posterior wall of the vestibule, there are five openings of semicircular canals.

D. On the anterior wall of the vestibule, there is a large opening communicating with the scala tympani.

19. About the bony semicircular canals, which of the following is **false**? (   )

A. Totally we have six bony crus.

B. The anterior one is also known as superior semicircular canal.

C. The lateral one is also called as horizontal semicircular canal.

D. Totally we have three bony semicircular canals

20. About the cochlear duct, which of the following is **false**? (   )

A. It is a spirally arranged canal.

B. It is filled with endolymph.

C. It has three walls.

D. The spiral organ is situated on the vestibular membrane.

21. About the osseous spiral lamina, which of the following is **false**? (   )

A. It is a bony structure.

B. It projects out from the modiolus.

C. It is helpful in dividing the scala vestibuli and the scala tympani.

D. It contains the spiral organs.

22. About the utricle, which of the following is **false**? (　　)

A. It lies in the vestibule.

B. On its posterior wall, there are four openings of the membranous semicircular ducts.

C. There is communicating duct located between utricle and saccule.

D. It contains macula utriculi.

23. About the semicircular ducts, which of the following is **false**? (　　)

A. They lie in the bony semicircular canals.

B. We have three semicircular ducts.

C. The semicircular ducts are filled with perilymph.

D. They have ampullae with ampullary crests inside.

24. Which of the following is **false**? (　　)

A. The macula utriculi can receive the linear acceleration stimulation.

B. The ampullary crests can receive the angular acceleration stimulation.

C. The spiral organ is the receptor of auditory sensation.

D. The macula sacculi can receive the rotation stimulation.

25. About the internal acoustic meatus, which of the following is **not** true? (　　)

A. It is located within the petrous part of the temporal bone.

B. There are facial nerve and vagus nerve located inside the internal acoustic meatus.

C. It communicates with the cranial cavity through internal acoustic pore.

D. The blood vessels of the labyrinth pass the internal acoustic meatus.

Ⅱ. Double choices (Choose the two best answers among the following choices, and write down the corresponding letters in bracket)

1. About theauricle, which ones of the following are **false**? (　　)

A. It projects from the side of the head.

B. It has bony framework.

C. It is composed of a thin plate of elastic fibrocartilage and covered by skin.

D. The auricular lobule is composed of fibrous and adipose tissue.

E. Its anterolateral surface shows irregular convex.

2. About theexternal acoustic meatus, which ones of the following are **false**? (　　)

A. It extends from the external acoustic pore to the tympanic membrane.

B. It is about 2.1 - 2.5 cm in length.

C. Its posterosuperior wall is longer than anteroinferior wall.

D. It comprises cartilaginous part and bony part.

E. There is no cartilage inside the wall of this meatus.

3. About the external acoustic meatus, which ones of the following are true? (　　)

    A. Its internal lumen is covered by mucous membrane.

    B. There is no sebaceous gland in the subcutaneous tissue of this meatus.

    C. Its lateral 1/3 is termed cartilaginous part.

    D. Its posterosuperior wall is longer than anteroinferior wall.

    E. Its internal lumen is covered by skin.

4. About the tympanic membrane, which ones of the following are **false**? (　　)

    A. It is triangle in appearance.

    B. It separates the middle ear from the external acoustic meatus.

    C. It forms an angle of 45 degrees with the floor of the meatus.

    D. Its lateral surface is covered by mucous membrane.

    E. It is composed of three layers.

5. About the tympanic membrane, which ones of the following are correct? (　　)

    A. It is rectangle in appearance.

    B. It separates the middle ear from the external acoustic meatus.

    C. It forms an angle of 45 degrees with the roof of the meatus.

    D. It is composed of two layers.

    E. Malleus is attached to the medial surface of the tympanic membrane.

6. Which ones of the following statements about the tympanic membrane are right? (　　)

    A. The umbo is located on the center of the membrane.

    B. The flaccid part is devoid of mucous membrane.

    C. Its skin is continuous with that of the external acoustic meatus.

    D. The flaccid part is thicker than the tense part.

    E. It has muscular layer.

7. About the tympanic membrane, which ones of the following are **not** true? (　　)

    A. Cuticular layer is the outer layer.

    B. Mucous layer is the inner layer.

    C. Fibrous layer is the intermediate layer.

    D. Muscular layer is the intermediate layer.

    E. The flaccid part accounts for most of the membrane.

8. About the tympanic cavity, which ones of the following are **false**? (　　)

    A. It is an irregular fluid-filled space.

    B. It possesses six walls.

    C. It lies between the tympanic membrane and the lateral wall of the inner ear.

    D. There are auditory ossicles inside the tympanic cavity.

    E. The anterior wall is called jugular wall.

9. About the tympanic cavity, which ones of the following are true? (　　)

    A. It is an irregular fluid-filled space.

    B. It is located inside the frontal bone.

C. It communicates with the nasopharynx anteriorly.

D. There are four auditory ossicles inside the tympanic cavity.

E. It communicates with the mastoid cells posteriorly.

10. Which ones of the following structures belong to the medial wall of the tympanic cavity? (   )

A. Pyramidal eminence

B. Fenestra vestibuli

C. Second tympanic membrane

D. Opening of the mastoid antrum

E. Auditory tube

11. The fenestra vestibuli is closed by (   ).

A. tympanic membrane

B. second tympanic membrane

C. base of stapes

D. annular ligament

E. spiral membrane

12. About the auditory tube, which ones of the following are **incorrect**? (   )

A. It isa channel through which the tympanic cavity communicates with nasopharynx.

B. It has two portions: the cartilaginous portion and bony portion.

C. It is approximately 3.5 – 4 cm long.

D. In childhood, the auditory tube is relatively longer than that in adult.

E. It begins in the posterior wall of the tympanic cavity and passes forward.

13. About the inner ear, which ones of the following are **incorrect**? (   )

A. It lies in the squamous portion of the temporal bone.

B. It consists of two parts: the bony labyrinth and membranous labyrinth.

C. The membranous labyrinth is composed of a series of membranous sacs and ducts.

D. The membranous labyrinth is filled with endolymph.

E. The bony labyrinth is composed of spongy bone.

14. The bony semicircular canals include the following canals **except** (   ).

A. anterior semicircular canal

B. lateral semicircular canal

C. medial semicircular canal

D. inferior semicircular canal

E. posterior semicircular canal

15. About the labyrinth, which ones of the following are **incorrect**? (   )

A. The cochlear spiral canal is a bony structure.

B. The cochlear duct is a membranous structure.

C. The cochlear duct is filled with perilymph.

D. The scala vestibuli and the scala tympani are filled with endolymph.

　　E. There are nerves and vessels inside the modiolus.

Ⅲ. Fill the blanks (Fill the most appropriate words in the blanks)

1. The vestibulocochlear organ is divided into three parts: _____ , _____ and

　　_____ .

2. The internal ear can receive two types of stimuli: _____ and _____ .

3. The middle ear consists of _____ , _____ and _____ .

4. The fenestra cochlea is closed by _____ .

5. The bony labyrinth is composed of _____ , _____ and _____ .

6. The three bony semicircular canals are _____ , _____ and _____ .

7. The linear acceleration or deceleration stimulation can be received by _____ and

　　_____ .

8. The membranous labyrinth inside the vestibule include _____ and _____ .

9. The structures located on the medial wall of the tympanic cavity include _____ ,

　　_____ and _____ .

10. The membranous labyrinth is filled with _____ .

11. The space between bony and membranous labyrinth is filled with _____ .

12. The spiral organ is situated on _____ .

13. The fenestra vestibuli is closed by _____ and _____ .

14. The tympanic cavity communicates with the nasopharynx through _____ .

15. The six wall of the tympanic cavity are _____ , _____ , _____ ,

　　_____ , _____ and _____ .

Ⅳ. Answer questions briefly

1. Please briefly describe the features and subdivisions of the external acoustic meatus.

2. Please briefly describe the six walls of the tympanic cavity.

3. Please briefly describe the elements of the middle ear.

4. Please describe the composition of the bony labyrinth.

5. Please describe the composition of the membranous labyrinth.

Ⅴ. Answer questions in detail

1. Please describe the six walls of the tympanic cavity and the communication of the

　　tympanic cavity.

2. Please describe the composition and function of the labyrinth.

3. Please describe the first pathway of the conduction of sound.

Ⅵ. Problems in life

1. How can you tell the direction of a sound?

2. Why does your voice sound different on a tape recording?

3. Why do we eventually stop hear a clock ticking?

Part 5　The Nervous System

Chapter 16　The Spinal Cord

I . **Single choice (Choose the best answer among the following four choices, and write down the corresponding letter in bracket)**

1. About the neuron, which one is **false**? (　　)

   A. Each neuron possesses a body and two types of processes

   B. Neuron contains one or more dendrites

   C. Neuron contains an axon

   D. Neuron has no nucleus

2. About the cell body of neuron, which one is **false**? (　　)

   A. It serves as metabolic center.

   B. It consists of a large pale nucleus and cytoplasm.

   C. It does not contain Nissl body.

   D. It varies in size and shape.

3. The axon (　　).

   A. terminates at the axon hillock

   B. comprises numerous synaptic vesicles

   C. branches repeatedly in a tree-like manner

   D. is also called nerve

4. About the neuroglia, which one is **false**? (　　)

   A. Neuroglia cells outnumber neurons in the CNS 10 : 1.

   B. Microglia are modified macrophages.

   C. Microglia are smaller and have fewer branching processes.

   D. The astrocytes have many radiating processes.

5. About nerve fibers, which one is **false**? (　　)

   A. Oligodendrocytes form myelin in central nervous system.

   B. Schwann cells form myelin in peripheral nerves.

   C. The longer processes of the neurons are termed nerve fibers.

   D. Nerve fibers are grouped into bundles to form the nerve.

6. The lower end of the spinal cord in adult is at the level of (　　).

A. lower border of the 12th thoracic vertebral body

B. upper border of the 1st lumbar vertebral body

C. lower border of the 1st lumbar vertebral body

D. upper border of the 2nd lumbar vertebral body

7. In adult, T_6 spinal segment is located at the level of vertebra (   ).

   A. T_4

   B. T_6

   C. T_8

   D. T_{10}

8. The posterior funiculus of spinal cord contains (   ).

   A. posterior spinocerebellar tract

   B. lateral spinothalamic tract

   C. fasciculus gracilis

   D. lateral corticospinal tract

9. Concerning the spinal cord, which one is **false**? (   )

   A. The spinal cord is located in the vertebral canal.

   B. The spinal cord extends from the foramen magnum.

   C. The spinal cord continues with the medulla oblongata.

   D. Its diameters are equal at various levels.

10. Which of the following statements about the spinal cord is **incorrect**? (   )

   A. The grey matter contains enormous number of neurons.

   B. The white matter is composed of myelinated and unmyelinated nerve fibers.

   C. The spinal cord consists of five external segments.

   D. Between the anterior and posterior horns is the intermediate zone.

11. The cervical enlargement is located at (   ).

   A. $C_4 - T_1$

   B. $C_6 - T_1$

   C. $C_8 - T_1$

   D. $C_1 - C_4$

12. The lumbosacral enlargement is situated at (   ).

   A. $L_1 - S_5$

   B. $L_1 - S_3$

   C. $L_3 - S_4$

   D. $S_2 - S_4$

13. In the transverse section, the spinal cord (   ).

   A. consists of the gray matter and the white matter

   B. has the lateral horn

   C. has the same size grey matter

   D. has twelve laminas

14. About the gray matter of the spinal cord, which one is **false**? (   )

   A. It contains neurons and neuroglial cells.

   B. It is an "H" shaped structure.

   C. It only contains sensory and motor nuclei.

   D. It has anterior horn, intermediate zone and posterior horn.

15. The nuclei in the anterior horn contain (   ).

   A. two main types of neuron

   B. nucleus proprius and nucleus thoracicus

   C. sacral parasympathetic nucleus

   D. α – motor neuron, γ – motor neuron and Renshaw cell

16. The intermediolateral nucleus (   ).

   A. constitutes the base of the lateral horn

   B. begins in the lower portion of C_6

   C. terminates caudally on L_3

   D. sends out parasympathetic fibers

17. The parasympathetic nucleus (   ).

   A. is found along the lateral surface in segments S_2, S_3 and S_4

   B. is situated in the white matter

   C. sends out the parasympathetic postganglionic fibers

   D. is found all the segments in spinal cord

18. The nuclei in the posterior horn contain (   ).

   A. nucleus dorsalis of Clarke

   B. sympathetic nucleus

   C. parasympathetic nucleus

   D. intermediomedial nucleus

19. The nucleus proprius (   ).

   A. is located in the Lamina I

   B. is located in Laminas III and IV

   C. is related to discriminating tactile

   D. conveys subconscious proprioceptive impulses to the cerebellum

20. About the spinal laminas, which of the following is true? (   )

   A. There are twelve laminas altogether.

   B. Laminas III and IV are referred to the nucleus proprius.

   C. Lamina IX is around the central canal.

   D. Lamina I corresponds to substantia gelatinosa.

21. About the white matter in the spinal cord, which one is **false**? (   )

   A. The spinal white matter surrounds the gray matter.

   B. It contains the ascending, descending tracts and propriospinal tracts.

   C. The tracts within the funiculi are all sensory fibers.

    D. It has anterior, lateral and posterior funiculi.

22. The fasciculus gracilis (   ).

    A. contains the fibers from sacral, lumbar and lower eight thoracic segments

    B. terminates upon the nuclei cuneatus

    C. conducts impulses of pain and temperature

    D. conducts impulses of pressure

23. The fasciculus cuneatus (   ).

    A. contains the fibers from upper four thoracic and cervical segments

    B. terminates upon the nuclei gracilis

    C. conducts impulses of pain and temperature

    D. conducts impulses of pressure

24. The posterior spinocerebellar tract (   ).

    A. is situated along the anterolateral periphery of the spinal cord

    B. arises from the ipsilateral dorsal nucleus

    C. descends through spinal cord to the medulla oblongata

    D. conveys conscious proprioceptive impulses

25. The spinothalamic tract (   ).

    A. is a long descending tract

    B. conveys the pain and thermal sense

    C. includes posterior and anterior spinothalamic tracts

    D. passes through the brain stem and ends directly in the cortex

26. The anterior spinothalamic tract (   ).

    A. arises from the nucleus proprius

    B. crosses in the anterior gray commissure

    C. descends contralaterally anterior to the lateral spinothalamic tract

    D. conveys conscious proprioceptive impulses

27. The long descending tracts do **not** (   ).

    A. administrate the somatic movement

    B. control the visceral innervation

    C. adjust the modification of the muscle tone

    D. arise from the spinal cord

28. The corticospinal tract (   ).

    A. arises from the spinal cord

    B. terminates in the cortex

    C. reaches the ipsilateral spinal cord

    D. is long descending fibers

29. About the lateral corticospinal tract, which is **false**? (   )

    A. It decussates in the medulla oblongata.

    B. It descends medially to the posterior spinocerebellar tract in the spinal cord.

C. It extends to the most caudal part of the spinal cord.

D. It extends only to the upper thoracic spinal segments.

30. About the anterior corticospinal tract, which is correct? (　　)

A. It occupies all over the spinal cord.

B. It extends to the most caudal part of the spinal cord.

C. It extends only to the upper thoracic spinal segments.

D. It mediates the extensor muscles.

31. The typical reflex arc does **not** contain (　　).

A. receptor

B. afferent neuron

C. efferent neuron

D. synapse

32. The synapse does **not** contain (　　).

A. presynaptic element

B. postsynaptic element

C. synaptic cleft

D. gap junction

33. About the classification of the neuron, which is **wrong**? (　　)

A. It only contains the sensory and motor neurons.

B. It can be classified by the size of the neurons.

C. It can be classified by the number of their processes.

D. It can be classified by the chemicals in the neurons.

34. The functions of the spinal cord is **not** to (　　).

A. convey afferent impulses

B. conduct efferent impulses

C. control the reflex

D. control the blood pressure

35. The patient with hemisection of the spinal cord may **not** have (　　).

A. ipsilateral lower motor neuron paralysis the segments of the lesion

B. ipsilateral upper motor neuron paralysis below the level of the lesion

C. ipsilateral loss of proprioceptive sense

D. ipsilateral loss of pain and temperature sense below one or two segments at the injured level

Ⅱ. Double choices(Choose the two best answers among the following choices, and write down the corresponding letters in bracket)

1. Which ones of the following are the neuroglia? (　　)

A. Astrocyte

B. Oligodendrocyte

    C. Renshaw cells

    D. α - motor neuron

    E. γ - motor neuron

2. About the neuron, which ones are correct? (　　　)

    A. Each neuron possesses a nucleated cell body and processes.

    B. They can form the myelin.

    C. The neurons outnumber neuroglial cells in CNS 10 : 1.

    D. The terminal segment of axon comprises numerous synaptic vesicles.

    E. The neuron does not contain Nissl body.

3. About the neuroglia, which ones are **false**? (　　　)

    A. The neuroglial cells involve the myelin formation.

    B. Ependymal cell is a type of neuroglia.

    C. Schwann cells are not the neuroglia

    D. Oligodendrocytes are modified macrophages.

    E. Astrocytes are neuroectodermal in origin.

4. The two enlargements in spinal cord comprise (　　　).

    A. cervical enlargement

    B. thoracic enlargement

    C. lumbosacral enlargement

    D. sacral enlargement

    E. coccygeal enlargement

5. The nuclei in the intermediate zone contain (　　　).

    A. substantia gelatinosa

    B. nucleus thoracicus

    C. sacral parasympathetic nucleus

    D. intermediomedial nucleus

    E. nucleus proprius

6. The nuclei in the posterior horn contain (　　　).

    A. substantia gelatinosa

    B. nucleus thoracicus

    C. sacral parasympathetic nucleus

    D. intermediomedial nucleus

    E. intermediolateral nucleus

7. About the nucleus thoracicus, which ones are correct? (　　　)

    A. It is situated in the medial portion of the base of the posterior horn.

    B. The nucleus thoracicus is located in Laminas Ⅶ.

    C. It receives the collateral branches of the primary efferent fibers.

    D. The axons contributed fibers to the posterior spinothalamic tracts.

    E. The nucleus thoracicus is located in Laminas Ⅲ and Ⅳ.

8. The long ascending tracts (   ).

   A. carry motor impulse from the brain to the spinal cord

   B. contain the fasciculus gracilis and fasciculus cuneatus

   C. carry sensory impulse from the spinal cord to the suprasegmental structures

   D. control the pain and thermal sense

   E. convey subconscious proprioceptive impulses to the cerebrum

9. About the long descending tracts, which ones are correct? (   )

   A. They are concerned with somatic movement, visceral innervation and modification of muscle tone.

   B. They mostly arise from the cerebral cortex or brain stem.

   C. The tectospinal tract play significant role in moderation of muscle tone and visceral activities.

   D. The rubrospinal tract is to increase the extensor muscle tone.

   E. The reticulospinal tract mediates the visual and auditory stimuli.

10. About the functions of the spinal cord, which ones are **false**? (   )

   A. It is to convey afferent impulses.

   B. It is to conduct efferent impulses.

   C. It is related to stretch reflex.

   D. It functions in maintaining equilibrium and controlling posture.

   E. It can coordinate subconscious contraction of skeletal muscles.

Ⅲ. Fill the blanks (Fill the most appropriate words in the blanks)

1. The central nervous system includes _____ and _____.

2. The nervous tissue consists of _____ and _____.

3. The neuroglial cells contain _____, _____ and _____.

4. The spinal cord has two enlargements, including _____ and _____.

5. The spinal cord tapers gradually and becomes the conical end known as _____.

6. The condensation of pia mater around the spinal cord forms the _____.

7. On the transverse section, the spinal cord is divided into _____ and _____.

8. _____ traverses the center of the grey commissure in spinal cord.

9. The spinal white matter can be divided into _____, _____ and _____.

10. The posterior funiculus has two long ascending tracts, they are _____ and _____.

11. Three main types of neuron are distributed within the anterior horn, they are _____, _____ and _____.

12. Anterior to the grey commissure is a bundle of transverse fibers, called _____.

13. In spinal cord, the structure around the central canal is the _____.

14. The cervical enlargement is situated from _____ to _____.

15. The lumbosacral enlargement is situated from _____ to _____.

16. In Laminas Ⅲ and Ⅳ, _____ is the main nucleus.

17. The corticospinal tract arises from the _____, descends through the _____ and _____.

18. The principle functions of the spinal cord are to _____ and _____.

19. The neurons aggregated group or cluster according to their functions in CNS are called _____.

20. The neurons aggregated group or cluster according to their functions in PNS are called _____.

Ⅳ. Answer questions briefly

1. Please describe the organization of the nervous system.

2. Please describe the reflex and reflex arc.

3. What is the difference between nucleus and ganglion?

4. What are the tracts in the white matter?

5. What are the nuclei in the posterior horn?

6. Please describe the long descending tracts in white matter.

7. Please describe the long ascending tracts in white matter.

8. What are the functions of the spinal cord?

Ⅴ. Answer questions in detail

1. Please describe the location and external features of the spinal cord.

2. Please describe the corticospinal tract and its functions.

Ⅵ. Problems in life

Have you heard the spinal hemisection and Brown-Sequard syndrome?

Chapter 17　The Brain Stem

Ⅰ. **Single choice（Choose the best answer among the following four choices, and write down the corresponding letter in bracket）**

1. The brainstem is formed by (　　).

    A. medulla oblongata, pons and cerebellum

    B. medulla oblongata, pons and thalamus

    C. pons, cerebellum and thalamus

    D. medulla oblongata, pons and midbrain

2. The rostral boundary of the brain stem is (　　).

    A. optic tract

    B. oculomotor nerve

    C. optic chiasma

    D. optic nerve

3. Which of the following nerves lies between the pyramid and olive? (　　)

    A. Glossopharyngeal nerve

    B. Vagus nerve

    C. Accessory nerve

    D. Hypoglossal nerve

4. Which nerve emerges from the junction of the basilar part of the pons and middle cerebellar peduncle? (　　)

    A. Trigeminal nerve

    B. Abducent nerve

    C. Facial nerve

    D. Vestibulocochlear nerve

5. In rhomboid fossa, a ridge on each side of the median sulcus is (　　).

    A. sulcus limitans

    B. medial eminence

    C. vagal triangle

    D. vestibular area

6. The rhomboid fossa is divided into pontine and medullary parts by (　　).

    A. bulbopontine sulcus

    B. medial sulcus

    C. sulcus limitans

    D. striae medullares

7. The nerve that emerges from the dorsal surface of brain stem is (　　).

A. oculomotor nerve

B. trochlear nerve

C. trigeminal nerve

D. hypoglossal nerve

8. Which of the following is the general somatic motor nucleus in the brain stem?
   (   )

   A. Nucleus of oculomotor nerve

   B. Accessory nucleus of oculomotor nerve

   C. Nucleus of facial nerve

   D. Nucleus ambiguus

9. Which of the following belongs to the special visceral motor nucleus? (   )

   A. Spinal nucleus of trigeminal nerve

   B. Pontine nucleus of trigeminal nerve

   C. Motor nucleus of trigeminal nerve

   D. Mesencephalic nucleus of trigeminal nerve

10. Which of the following belongs to the special somatic sensory nucleus? (   )

    A. Nucleus of hypoglossal nerve

    B. Nucleus of facial nerve

    C. Nucleus ambiguous

    D. Cochlear nucleus

11. The nucleus which gives fiber that innervates the smooth muscles and glands is
    (   ).

    A. Nucleus of trigeminal nerve

    B. Nucleus of trochlear nerve

    C. Dorsal nucleus of vagus nerve

    D. Nucleus of oculomotor nerve

12. Which of the following nuclei is located beneath the facial colliculus? (   )

    A. Nucleus of facial nerve

    B. Nucleus of abducent nerve

    C. Motor nucleus of trigeminal nerve

    D. Nucleus ambiguous

13. Which structure is **not** located in the rhomboid fossa? (   )

    A. Median sulcus

    B. Sulcus limitans

    C. Basilar sulcus

    D. Facial colliculus

14. Which of the following cranial nerves does **not** attach to the pons? (   )

    A. Trochlear nerve

    B. Trigeminal nerve

C. Abducent nerve

D. Facial nerve

15. Which nucleus of cranial nerves are concerned with taste sensation? (   )

    A. Vestibular nucleus

    B. Nucleus ambiguous

    C. Dorsal nucleus of vagus nerve

    D. Nucleus of solitary tract

16. Which structure lies on the dorsal surface of the brain stem? (   )

    A. Pyramid

    B. Basilar part of pons

    C. Cerebral peduncle

    D. Superior colliculus

17. The mesencephalic aqueduct communicates directly with (   ).

    A. lateral ventricles

    B. lateral and third ventricles

    C. third and fourth ventricles

    D. fourth ventricle and the central canal

18. The fibers from the nucleus ambiguus join in (   ).

    A. glossopharyngeal nerve, vagus nerve, hypoglossal nerve

    B. hypoglossal nerve, accessory nerve and vagus nerve

    C. vagus nerve, glossopharyngeal nerve and accessory nerve

    D. facial nerve, glossopharyngeal nerve and vagus nerve

19. About the decussation of medial lemniscus, which of the following is correct?

    (   )

    A. It is formed by the crossing fibers of motor tract

    B. It lies above the decussation of pyramid

    C. It lies at the level of the facial colliculus

    D. It is formed by the crossing fibers of spinal lemniscus

20. Which of the following nuclei lies in the medulla oblongata? (   )

    A. Motor nucleus of trigeminal nerve

    B. Nucleus of facial nerve

    C. Abducent nucleus

    D. Inferior salivatory nucleus

21. The nerve which attaches to the bulbopontine sulcus is (   ).

    A. oculomotor nerve

    B. abducent nerve

    C. hypoglossal nerve

    D. vagus nerve

22. Trigeminal lemniscus arises from (   ).

A. trigeminal ganglion

B. spinal ganglion

C. pontine and spinal nuclei of trigeminal nerve

D. motor nucleus of trigeminal nerve

23. Which of the following is **not** related to the reticular formation of brain stem? ( )

A. Optic center

B. Cardiovascular controlling center

C. Respiratory center

D. Vomiting center

24. The fibers of lateral lemniscus arise from ( ).

A. contralateral cochlear nucleus

B. ipsilateral cochlear nucleus

C. bilateral cochlear nucleus

D. bilateral vestibular and cochlear nucleus

25. Which structure forms the trapezoid body? ( )

A. Fibers from the trigeminal lemniscus

B. Fibers from the medial lemniscus

C. Fibers from the lateral lemniscus

D. Fibers from the cochlear nucleus

26. Which of the following is **not** a structure of the reticular formation? ( )

A. Rapheal nucleus

B. Lateral reticular nucleus

C. Olivary nucleus

D. Mesencephalic reticular nucleus

27. The long descending tract in the brain stem is ( ).

A. Medial lemniscus

B. Lateral lemniscus

C. Trigeminal lemniscus

D. Pyramidal tract

28. The pretectal nucleus is situated at ( ).

A. midbrain

B. pons

C. rhomboid fossa

D. medulla oblongata

29. Which of the following is on anterior surface of medulla oblongata? ( )

A. Interpeduncular fossa

B. Basilar sulcus

C. Olive

　　D. Gracile tubercle

30. Which of the followings is **not** related to the hearing transmission? (　　)

　　A. Cochlear nucleus

　　B. Superior olivary nucleus

　　C. Lateral lemniscus

　　D. Superior colliculus

Ⅱ. Double choices(Choose the two best answers among the following choices, and write down the corresponding letters in bracket)

1. Which ones of the following belong to the special somatic sensory nuclei? (　　)

　　A. Hypoglossal nucleus

　　B. Spinal nucleus of trigeminal nerve

　　C. Facial nucleus

　　D. Vestibular nucleus

　　E. Cochlear nucleus

2. Medial lemniscus arises from (　　).

　　A. gracile nucleus

　　B. cuneate nucleus

　　C. pontine nucleus

　　D. spinal nucleus of trigeminal nerve

　　E. motor nucleus of trigeminal nerve

3. The eminences on the dorsum of the midbrain are (　　).

　　A. superior colliculus

　　B. inferior colliculus

　　C. facial colliculus

　　D. pyramid

　　E. olive

4. Which ones of the following arise from the midbrain? (　　)

　　A. Oculomotor nerve

　　B. Optic nerve

　　C. Trochlear nerve

　　D. Trigeminal nerve

　　E. Facial nerve

5. Nucleus ambiguus does **not** contribute to (　　).

　　A. facial nerve

　　B. glossopharyngeal nerve

　　C. vagus nerve

　　D. accessory nerve

　　E. hypoglossal nerve

6. Which nuclei are **not** related to the facial nerve? (   )

A. Superior salivatory nucleus

B. Inferior salivatory nucleus

C. Nuclei of solitary tract

D. Nuclei of facial nerve

E. Spinal nuclei of trigeminal nerve

7. Thenon-cranial nuclei in the midbrain include (   ).

A. nucleus ceruleus

B. gracile nucleus

C. cuneate nucleus

D. red nucleus

E. substantia nigra

8. Which ones of the following about the inferior olivary nucleus complex are **incorrect**?

(   )

A. It is located deep to the olive.

B. It is divided into 3 nuclei.

C. It receives fibers from the superior olivary nucleus

D. It receives fibers from the cerebellar nucleus.

E. The efferent fibers enter the inferior cerebellar peduncle.

9. The structures on anterior surface of pons include (   ).

A. cerebral peduncle

B. basilar sulcus

C. medial sulcus

D. sulcus limitans

E. trigeminal nerve

10. The structures on anterior surface of midbrain include (   ).

A. cerebral peduncle

B. oculomotor nerve

C. trochlear nerve

D. trigeminal nerve

E. superior colliculus

Ⅲ. Fill the blanks (Fill the most appropriate words in the blanks)

1. The brainstem consists of _____ , _____ and _____ from below upwards.

2. At the lower angle of the fourth ventricle, the fasciculus gracilis ends in _____.
Lateral and adjacent to it, there is another swelling, it is _____.

3. The median groove on the ventral surface of the pons is _____.

4. The nerves emerge from the bulbopontine sulcus are _____ , _____ , and

_____ .

5. Medial eminence is bounded laterally by _____ , medially by _____ .

6. The _____ divide the rhomboid fossa into pontine and medullary parts.

7. The structures deep to the facial colliculus are _____ and _____ .

8. Below the striae medullares on each side of the median sulcus, there are two triangular areas, medial one is _____ , lateral one is _____ .

9. Two longitudinal columns of nerve fibers on ventral surface of the midbrain are _____ _____ . A deep depression bounded by them is _____ .

10. On the dorsal surface of the midbrain there are 2 pairs of eminence, they are _____ _____ the _____ and _____ .

11. The motor root of trigeminal nerve arises from the _____ .

12. The nucleus ambiguus provides the special visceral efferent fibers for _____ , _____ and _____ nerves.

13. The general visceral motor nuclei include _____ , _____ , _____ , and _____ .

14. The special somatic sensory nuclei include _____ and _____ .

15. Axons from gracile and cuneate nuclei form the _____ .

16. In midbrain, _____ is a lamina of gray matter containing pigmented nerve cells.

17. The spinothalamic lemniscus is composed of _____ and _____ .

18. In transverse section of the midbrain the substantia nigra separates _____ from the _____ .

19. The axons of the spinal and pontine nucleus of trigeminal nerve successively cross the median plane to form the _____ .

20. Rostrolateral to the gracile and cuneate tubercles, a thick round ridge is _____ .

IV. Answer questions briefly

1. Please briefly describe the origin, termination and function of the medial lemniscus.

2. Please briefly describe the boundaries and external features of the rhomboid fossa.

3. In brain stem, which nuclei give off the fibers to innervate the muscles of eye?

4. In brain stem, which nuclei are related to the facial nerve?

5. In brain stem, which nuclei are related to the sense and movement of tongue?

6. Please briefly describe the reticular formation (the concept, the main function).

7. Please briefly describe the external features of the midbrain.

8. Which nuclei in the brain stem are related to the movement of skeletal muscles in head and neck?

V. Answer questions in detail

1. Please describe the important structures on the horizontal section at the middle part

of olive.

2. Please describe the important structures on the horizontal section at the level of facial colliculus.

3. Please describe the important structures on the horizontal section at the inferior colliculus of the midbrain.

Ⅵ. Problems in life

What is a "broken neck"?

Chapter 18   The Cerebellum

Ⅰ. **Single choice (Choose the best answer among the following four choices, and write down the corresponding letter in bracket)**

1. The cerebellum is located in (   ).
   A. the anterior cranial fossa
   B. the middle cranial fossa
   C. the posterior cranial fossa
   D. the hypophysial fossa

2. The central constricted area of the cerebellum is called (   ).
   A. the tonsils
   B. the vermis
   C. the hemisphere
   D. the nodule

3. The flocculonodular lobe is also called (   ).
   A. thevestibulocerebellum
   B. the spinocerebellum
   C. the cerebrocerebellum
   D. the paleocerebellum

4. Which of the following does **not** belong to the vermis? (   )
   A. The tonsils
   B. The pyramid of vermis
   C. The uvula of vermis
   D. The nodule

5. The tonsils belong to (   ).
   A. the flocculonodular lobe
   B. the anterior lobe
   C. the vermis
   D. the hemispheres

6. About the paleocerebellum, which statement is correct? (   )
   A. It is consisted of the anterior lobe and the rostral part of the inferior vermis.
   B. It is concerned with coordinating muscular activities.
   C. It receives the fibers from the dentate nucleus.
   D. It is called the archicerebellum.

7. Which of the following does **not** belong to cerebellar nuclei? (   )
   A. The fastigial nucleus

    B. The globose nucleus

    C. The red nucleus

    D. The dentate nucleus

8. The superior cerebellar peduncle is called (   ).

    A. the restiform body

    B. the brachium conjunctivum

    C. the brachium pontis

    D. the vermis

9. The middle cerebellar peduncle is composed almost by (   ).

    A. the vestibular nerve

    B. the posterior spinocerebellar tract

    C. the anterior spinocerebellar tract

    D. the pontocerebellar fibers

10. Which of the following structures receives the pontocerebellar fibers? (   )

    A. The flocculonodular lobe

    B. The anterior lobe

    C. The middle lobe

    D. The posterior lobe

11. Which of the following associates to the adjustment of muscular tonicity? (   )

    A. The archicerebellum

    B. The paleocerebellum

    C. The neocerebellum

    D. The cerebrocerebellum

12. Which nucleus receives the fibers from the cerebrocerebellum? (   )

    A. The fastigial nucleus

    B. The globose nucleus

    C. The emboliform nucleus

    D. The dentate nucleus

13. Which of the following nuclei receives the fibers from the flocculonodular lobe? (   )

    A. the fastigial nucleus

    B. the red nucleus

    C. the dentate nucleus

    D. the pontine nucleus

14. The structure related to the coordination of muscular activities is (   ).

    A. the flocculonodular lobe

    B. the vestibulocerebellum

    C. the spinocerebellum

    D. the pontocerebellum

15. Which function does **not** belong to cerebellum? (   )

    A. The maintaining of equilibrium

    B. The adjustment of muscular tonicity

    C. The coordination of muscular activities

    D. The voluntary movement of the skeletal muscles

II . **Double choices(Choose the two best answers among the following choices, and write down the corresponding letters in bracket)**

1. The cerebellum is (   ).

    A. inferior to the diencephalon

    B. posterior to occipital lobes of the cerebrum

    C. anterior to the medulla oblongata and pons

    D. separated from the cerebrum by the tentorium cerebelli

    E. connected with the brain stem by the cerebellar peduncles

2. Which ones of the following structures belong to cerebellar nuclei? (   )

    A. The fastigial nucleus

    B. The globose nucleus

    C. The lentiform nucleus

    D. The reticular nucleus

    E. The caudate nucleus

3. Which ones of the following projection fibers do **not** connect the cerebellum with the brain? (   )

    A. The superior cerebellar peduncle

    B. The middle cerebellar peduncle

    C. The inferior cerebellar peduncle

    D. The cerebral peduncle

    E. The pyramid

4. The fibers from the spinocerebellum project to (   ).

    A. the fastigial nucleus

    B. the globose nucleus

    C. the lentiform nucleus

    D. the emboliform nucleus

    E. the dentate nucleus

5. Which ones of the following structures do **not** belong to cerebellar cortex? (   )

    A. The polymorphic layer

    B. The molecular layer

    C. The granular layer

    D. The Purkinje layer

    E. The pyramidal layer

Ⅲ. Fill the blanks (Fill the most appropriate words in the blanks)

1. The cerebellum consists of two _____ joined by _____.

2. The cerebellum is attached to the brain stem by three paired bundles of fibers called _____ , _____ and _____ .

3. The cerebellum can be divided into three lobes, they are _____ , _____ and _____ .

4. The central nuclei of the cerebellum are _____ , _____ , _____ and _____ .

5. The cerebellar cortex consist of three layers, they are _____ , _____ and _____ .

Ⅳ. Answer questions briefly

1. Please briefly describe the position and shape of the cerebellum.

2. Please briefly describe the cerebellar peduncles.

3. Please briefly describe the layers of the cerebellar cortex.

Ⅴ. Answer questions in detail

1. Please describe the central nuclei of the cerebellum and its fiber links with cerebellar cortex.

2. Please describe the lobe of cerebellum and their functions.

Ⅵ. Problems in life

1. Does the weight of brain increase after childhood?

2. Does the cerebellum take part in the learning and memory?

Chapter 19   The Diencephalon

I. **Single choice (Choose the best answer among the following four choices, and write down the corresponding letter in bracket)**

1. About the dorsal thalamus, which statement is **not** correct? (   )
   A. It is an oval structure below the midbrain.
   B. It consists of paired oval masses of most gray matter organized into nuclei.
   C. The masses are joined by the intermediate mass.
   D. It is separated from the hypothalamus by the hypothalamic sulcus.

2. Which of the following structures is located posterolaterally to the thalamus? (   )
   A. The hypothalamus
   B. The epithalamus
   C. The subthalamus
   D. The metathalamus

3. The structure belongs to the lateral nuclear group of the thalamus is (   ).
   A. the pulvinar
   B. the anterior tubercle
   C. the reticular nucleus
   D. the dorsomedial nucleus

4. Which of the following does **not** belong to the thalamus? (   )
   A. The pulvinar
   B. The ventral posterolateral nucleus
   C. The lateral geniculate nucleus
   D. The ventral posteromedial nucleus

5. The ventral posteromedial nucleus of the thalamus receives (   ).
   A. spinal lemniscus
   B. trigeminal lemniscus
   C. medial lemniscus
   D. lateral lemniscus

6. Which of the following does **not** belong to the hypothalamus (   ).
   A. the mammillary bodies
   B. the optic tracts
   C. the optic chiasma
   D. the pineal body

7. The ventral posterolateral nucleus of the thalamus receives (   ).
   A. the optic tract

B. the trigeminal lemniscus

C. the medial lemniscus

D. the lateral lemniscus

8. Which of the following nuclei receives trigeminothalamic tract? (   )

A. The ventral anterior nucleus

B. The ventral posteromedial nucleus

C. The ventral posterolateral nucleus

D. The ventral intermediate nucleus

9. Which of the following nuclei receives the spinothalamic tract? (   )

A. The ventral anterior nucleus

B. The ventral posteromedial nucleus

C. The ventral posterolateral nucleus

D. The ventral intermediate nucleus

10. The structure belongs to the epithalamus is (   ).

A. the optic chiasma

B. the pineal gland

C. the tuber cinereum

D. the papillary body

11. The nucleus belonging to the medial nucleus group is (   ).

A. the dorsomedial nucleus

B. the reticular nucleus

C. the anterior tubercle

D. the ventral posterior nucleus

12. The lateral geniculate body belongs to (   ).

A. the thalamus

B. the epithalamus

C. the subthalamus

D. the metathalamus

13. Which of the following nuclei receives the optic tract? (   )

A. The lateral geniculate nucleus

B. The medial geniculate nucleus

C. The pineal gland

D. The papillary body

14. Which of the following nuclei gives rise to the optic radiation? (   )

A. The lateral geniculate nucleus

B. The medial geniculate nucleus

C. The ventral posterolateral nucleus

D. The ventral intermediate nucleus

15. The medial geniculate nucleus receives (   ).

A. The fibers of the spinal lemniscus

B. The fibers of the trigeminal lemniscus

C. The fibers of the medial lemniscus

D. The fibers of the lateral lemniscus

16. Which of the following nuclei gives rise to the acoustic radiation? (   )

A. The lateral geniculate nucleus

B. The medial geniculate nucleus

C. The ventral posterolateral nucleus

D. The ventral intermediate nucleus

17. Which of the following functions does **not** belong to the hypothalamus? (   )

A. It control the activities of the central nervous system.

B. It is associated with feeling of rage.

C. It controls normal body temperature.

D. It regulates food intake through the feeding center.

18. The third ventricle, through the mesencephalic aqueduct, communicates with

(   ).

A. the right lateral ventricle

B. the second ventricle

C. the fourth ventricle

D. the left lateral ventricle

19. About the diencephalon, which statement is correct? (   )

A. Between the cerebullum and the hemispheres of the cerebrum

B. Only the epithalamic structures can be viewed

C. Exposes only the ventral surface of the diencephalon

D. Consists of six the thalami

20. The structure belongs to the metathalamus is (   ).

A. the pineal body

B. the medial geniculate body

C. the optic chiasma

D. the papillary body

Ⅱ. **Double choices(Choose the two best answers among the following choices, and write down the corresponding letters in bracket)**

1. The nuclei belonging to the specific thalamic nuclei are (   ).

A. the reticular nucleus

B. the ventral posterolateral nucleus

C. the lateral geniculate nucleus

D. the ventral posteromedial nucleus

E. the intralaminar nucleus

2. Which ones of the following fibers project to the ventral posteromedial nucleus?
   (   )
   A. The spinothalamic tract
   B. The trigeminal lemniscus
   C. The medial lemniscus
   D. The lateral lemniscus
   E. The optic tracts

3. Which ones of the following do **not** belong to the nonspecific thalamic nuclei? (   )
   A. The pulvinar
   B. The lateral geniculate nucleus
   C. The lateral dorsal nucleus
   D. The ventral posterolateral nucleus
   E. The dorsomedial nucleus

4. The nuclei projecting fibers to the general sensory area of cortex are (   ).
   A. the medial geniculate nucleus
   B. the ventral posterolateral nucleus
   C. the lateral geniculate nucleus
   D. the ventral posteromedial nucleus
   E. the intralaminar nucleus

5. Which ones of the following structures communicate with the third ventricle? (   )
   A. The lateral ventricle
   B. The second ventricle
   C. The fourth ventricle
   D. The subarachnoid space
   E. The central canal

Ⅲ. **Fill the blanks (Fill the most appropriate words in the blanks)**

1. The diencephalon consists of _____ , _____ , _____ , _____
   and _____ .
2. The thalamus masses are, by internal medullary lamina, divided into _____ ,
   _____ and _____ .
3. The thalamic nuclei, on the basis of phylogeny and function, may be classified into
   _____ , _____ , _____ and _____ .
4. The metathalamus includes _____ and _____ .
5. The epithalamus includes _____ , _____ , _____ and _____ .
6. The hypothalamus includes _____ , _____ , _____ , _____ ,
   _____ , _____ and _____ .

Ⅳ. **Answer questions briefly**

1. Please describe the nuclear groups of the thalamus.
2. Please describe the position and parts of the diencephalon .
3. Please describe the position of the metathalamus and its nuclei.

Ⅴ. **Answer questions in detail**

Please describe the specific thalamic nuclei of the dorsal thalamus and its functions.

Ⅵ. **Problems in life**

What is the difference between a concussion and a contusion?

Chapter 20　The Telencephalon

Ⅰ. **Single choice (Choose the best answer among the following four choices, and write down the corresponding letter in bracket)**

1. The lobe, in front of the lateral sulcus and the central sulcus at the dorsal lateral surface of the cerebral hemisphere, is called (　　).
   A. frontal lobe
   B. parietal lobe
   C. temporal lobe
   D. occipital lobe

2. The precentral gyrus is located in (　　).
   A. parietal lobe
   B. frontal lobe
   C. temporal lobe
   D. occipital lobe

3. The sulcus located in occipital lobe is (　　).
   A hippocampal sulcus
   B. calcarine sulcus
   C. lateral sulcus
   D. central sulcus

4. The lobe that can **not** be seen from the surface of cerebral hemisphere is (　　).
   A. frontal lobe
   B. occipital lobe
   C. temporal lobe
   D. insula lobe

5. The central sulcus is located (　　).
   A. between parietal lobe and temporal lobe
   B. between parietal lobe and occipital lobe
   C. in the medial side of the cerebral hemisphere
   D. between frontal lobe, parietal lobe and temporal lobe

6. The gyrus that belongs to the temporal lobe is (　　).
   A. parahippocampal gyrus
   B. straight gyrus
   C. lingual gyrus
   D. cingulate gyrus

7. Which of the following lobe does **not** belong to the limbic lobe? (　　)

A. Hippocampus

B. Dentate gyrus

C. Parahippocampal gyrus

D. Paracentral lobe

8. The cortical area for head and face in the first somatic motor area is located in
(   ).

A. superior part of precentral gyrus

B. middle part of precentral gyrus

C. inferior part of precentral gyrus

D. anterior part of paracentral lobe

9. Which is the **wrong** statement about the visual area? (   )

A. It is also called striate area.

B. It receives the fibers from medial geniculate body.

C. The occipital lobe above the calcarine sulcus receives the impulse from the upper
retina.

D. Damage to one-side visual area leads to the blindness in the contralateral field of
vision of both eyes.

10. The acoustic area is located in (   ).

A. angular gyrus

B. superior temporal gyrus

C. transverse temporal gyrus

D. parahippocampal gyrus

11. The damage to the angular gyrus will lead to (   ).

A. motor aphasia

B. agraphia

C. alexia

D. sensory aphasia

12. The eloquent cortex is located in (   ).

A. posterior part of the superior frontal gyrus

B. posterior part of the middle frontal gyrus

C. posterior part of the inferior frontal gyrus

D. anterior part of the inferior frontal gyrus

13. The somesthetic area is located in (   ).

A. the postcentral gyrus and the posterior part of paracentral lobule

B. precentral gyrus and the anterior part of paracentral lobule

C. superior parietal lobule

D. insular cortex

14. The structure that belongs to the paleocortex is (   ).

A. hippocampus

B. dentate gyrus

C. olfactory bulb

D. medial occipitotemporal gyrus

15. Which of the following structure does **not** belong to the basal nuclei? (   )

A. Caudate nucleus

B. Substantia nigra

C. Lenticular nucleus

D. Amygdala

16. Striatum includes (   ).

A. caudate nucleus and amygdala

B. lenticular nucleus and amygdala

C. lenticular nucleus and caudate nucleus

D. caudate nucleus and claustrum

17. The structure that belongs to the paleostriatum is (   ).

A. caudate nucleus

B. lentiform putamen

C. globus pallidus

D. claustrum

18. The inferior horn of the lateral ventricle is located in (   ).

A. occipital lobe

B. temporal lobe

C. parietal lobe

D. frontal lobe

19. The structure connecting lateral and third ventricles is called (   ).

A. interventricular foramina

B. mesencephalic aqueduct

C. lateral foramen

D. median aperture

20. The statement of the medulla of the cerebral hemisphere, which one is **not** true?
(   )

A. It is located in the deep part of cortex.

B. It is made up of nerve fibers that connect with the various parts of the cortex only.

C. It can be divided into association fiber, commissural fibers and projection fibers.

D. The association fibers connect with the various parts of the cortex in the same hemisphere only.

21. The short fibers associated with the adjacent cerebral gyrus is (   ).

A. superior longitudinal fasciculus

B. inferior longitudinal fasciculus

    C. arcuate fibers

    D. cingulum

22. The contact fibers that unite the frontal and anterior temporal lobes is (　　).

    A. uncinate fasciculus

    B. superior longitudinal fasciculus

    C. cingulum

    D. inferior longitudinal fasciculus

23. About the description of corpus callosum, which one is **incorrect**? (　　)

    A. Located in the bottom of fissura telodiencephalica.

    B. It can be divided intofour parts: rostrum, genu, trunk and splenium.

    C. It is the major transverse commissure connecting the cerebral hemisphere and roofs in the lateral ventricle.

    D. The fibers in corpus callosum connect the orbital cortex, frontal lobes wide neo-cortical area of the hemisphere and the bilateral cortical areas of the occipital lobes.

24. Which one of the following does **not** belong to the commissural fibers? (　　)

    A. Anterior commissure

    B. Fornix

    C. Fornical commissure

    D. Corpus callosum

25. About the position and shape of the internal capsule, which one is **incorrect**? (　　)

    A. It consists of an anterior limb, a genu and a posterior limb.

    B. It is located between the caudate nucleus and the lenticular nucleus.

    C. The anterior limb is bounded by the lenticular nucleus and dorsal thalamus.

    D. The dorsal thalamus is in the medial part of the internal capsule.

26. Which of the following parts does **not** belong to the posterior limb of internal capsule? (　　)

    A. Thalamolentiform part

    B. Superior lentiform part

    C. Sublentiform part

    D. Retrolentiform part

27. The fibers pass through the sublentiform part of the posterior limb of internal capsule is (　　).

    A. corticospinal tract

    B. corticorubral tract

    C. optic radiation

    D. middle thalamic radiation

28. Usually the damage to the posterior limb of internal capsule will **not** cause (　　).

    A. voluntary motor paralysis

  B. impairment of general sensation

  C. blindness

  D. deafness

29. The tract that includes the projection from the ventral posterior thalamic nucleus to the somesthetic area in the parietal lobe is (　　).

  A. central thalamic radiation

  B. corticospinal tract

  C. corticorubral tract

  D. optic radiation

30. The fibers that pass through the genu of internal capsule are called (　　).

  A. central thalamic radiation

  B. corticospinal tract

  C. corticonuclear tract

  D. optic radiation

Ⅱ. Double choices(Choose the two best answers among the following choices, and write down the corresponding letters in bracket)

1. The sulci located in the superolateral surface of the cerebral hemisphere are (　　).

  A. central sulcus

  B. parietooccipital sulcus

  C. lateral sulcus

  D. calcarine sulcus

  E. cingulate sulcus

2. The gyri located in frontal lobe are (　　).

  A. superior frontal gyrus

  B. precentral gyrus

  C. postcentral gyrus

  D. angular gyrus

  E. supramarginal gyrus

3. Hippocampal formation includes (　　).

  A. hippocampus

  B. parahippocampal gyrus

  C. uncus of Para hippocampal gyrus

  D. dentate gyrus

  E. cingulate gyrus

4. Gyri in limbic lobe does **not** include (　　).

  A. cingulate gyrus

  B. paraterminal gyrus

  C. Inferior frontal gyrus

　　D. lingual gyrus

　　E. parahippocampal gyrus

5. Which ones of the following statements regarding basal nucleus are correct? (　　)

　　A. In the white matter near the bottom of the brain

　　B. Consists of caudate nucleus, lentiform nucleus and amygdala

　　C. Lentiform nucleus located in the inner side of internal capsule

　　D. Lentiform nucleus can be divided into putamen and the globus pallidus

　　E. Striatum includes caudate nucleus and amygdala

6. Striatum consists of (　　).

　　A. lentiform nucleus

　　B. dorsal thalamus

　　C. caudate nucleus

　　D. claustrum

　　E. amygdala

7. Which ones of the following statements about the first somatic sensory area are **wrong**? (　　).

　　A. Located in postcentral gyrus and the posterior part of paracentral lobe

　　B. Receive the sensory fibers from the ventral anterior thalamic nucleus

　　C. The body is represented in this area is inverted, including head

　　D. The sensory is from contralateral half of body

　　E. The size of the cortical area for a particular part of the body is determined by the functional importance of the part and its need for sensitivity.

8. The structures that belong to the commissural fibers are (　　).

　　A. corpus callosum

　　B. fornix

　　C. fornical commissure

　　D. cingulum

　　E. uncinate fasciculus

9. Which ones of the following do **not** pass through the posterior limb of internal capsule? (　　)

　　A. Corticorubral tract

　　B. Corticospinal tract

　　C. Middle thalamic radiation

　　D. Corticonuclear tract

　　E. Anterior thalamic radiation

10. Which ones of the following statements are correct about the language area? (　　)

　　A. Motor language area occupies the posterior part of inferior frontal gurus.

　　B. Damage of the posterior part of middle frontal gyrus will cause motor aphasia.

　　C. Auditory language area is located in angular gyrus.

D. Damage of visual language area will cause alexia.

E. Language area must have located in the left hemisphere.

III. Fill the blanks (Fill the most appropriate words in the blanks)

1. The fissure separating the left and right cerebral hemispheres is _____. The fissure separating the cerebellum from the brain is _____.

2. The five lobes of cerebral hemispheres are _____, _____, _____, _____ and _____.

3. On the superolateral surface of the hemisphers, the main Gyri in the frontal lobe are _____, _____, _____ and _____.

4. The hippocampal formation includes _____ and _____.

5. The basal nuclei consist of _____, _____, _____ and _____.

6. The lentiform nucleus consists of _____ and _____. _____ is also called paleostriatum.

7. Lateral ventricles are divided into _____, _____, _____ and _____ four parts. The lateral ventricles communicate with the third ventricle through the _____.

8. The auditory area is located in _____. The visual area surrounds the _____.

9. Motor language area occupies the _____. Dysfunction of motor language area will cause _____.

10. Visual language area occupies the _____. The damage of visual language area will cause _____.

11. The medullary center is composed of three types of fibers, they are _____, _____ and _____.

12. On the median sagittal plane, from forward backward, the corpus callosum can be divided into four parts: _____, _____, _____ and _____.

13. The association fibers that connect the gyri in the same hemisphere are _____, _____, _____ and _____.

14. On the horizontal plane, the internal capsule consists of three parts: _____, _____ and _____.

15. The ascending tracts pass through the posterior limb of internal capsule are _____, _____ and _____.

IV. Answer questions briefly

1. What are the main sulci and gyri of temporal lobe?

2. What are the main sulci and gyri of the frontal lobe?

3. What are the commissural fibers?

4. Please describe the position and projection characteristics of the somatic motor area.

5. Please describe the limbic system.

6. What are the language centers of human beings?

7. What are the composition of basal ganglia?

V. Answer questions in detail

1. Please describe the position, shape and the main fibers pass through internal capsule.

2. Please describe the lateral ventricles in the brain.

VI. Problems in life

1. How much energy does the brain require during a two-hour exam?

2. How long can the brain be deprived of oxygen before it becomes damaged?

Chapter 21　The Nervous Pathways

I . **Single choice (Choose the best answer among the following four choices, and write down the corresponding letter in bracket)**

1. The second neurons of the superficial sensory pathway of trunk and limbs are located in (　　).

   A. lamina I , IV to VII of spinal cord

   B. lamina V to VIII of spinal cord

   C. gracile and cuneate nuclei

   D. ventroposterolateral nucleus of thalamus

2. The structure associated with the superficial sensory pathway of head and face is (　　).

   A. lamina I , IV to VII of spinal cord

   B. trigeminal ganglion

   C. ventroposterolateral nucleus of thalamus

   D. postcentral gyrus and posterior part of the paracentral lobule

3. The third neurons of the deep sensory pathway of the trunk and limbs are located in (　　).

   A. gracile and cuneate nuclei

   B. anterior nuclear group of thalamus

   C. ventroposteromedial nucleus of thalamus

   D. ventroposterolateral nucleus of thalamus

4. The structure independent of fine tactile of the upper limbs is (　　).

   A. spinal ganglia

   B. the fasciculus cuneatus

   C. the medial lemniscus

   D. ventroposteromedial nucleus of thalamus

5. About the description of the spinothalamic lemniscus, which one is correct? (　　)

   A. It comes from the thoracic nucleus of the spinal cord

   B. It comes from gracile and cuneate nuclei

   C. It is the fibers before they cross.

   D. It is the conduct of warm pain in contralateral trunk and limbs

6. The sensory pathways of the trunk and limbs consist of neurons of (　　).

   A. one order

   B. two orders

   C. three orders

　　D. four orders

7. The site where the fibers come from second neurons of the superficial sensory pathway of the trunk and limbs intersect is (　　).

　　A. spinal cord

　　B. medulla oblongata

　　C. pons

　　D. midbrain

8. The third neurons of the superficial sensory pathway of the trunk and limbs are located in (　　).

　　A. gracile and cuneate nuclei

　　B. lateral geniculate body

　　C. ventroposteromedial nucleus of thalamus

　　D. ventroposterolateral nucleus of thalamus

9. The site where the fibers come from second neurons of the superficial sensory pathway of the head and face intersect is (　　).

　　A. spinal cord

　　B. diencephalon

　　C. brain stem

　　D. midbrain

10. Which first neurons of the following are **not** spinal ganglia? (　　)

　　A. The superficial sensory pathway of the head and face

　　B. The superficial sensory pathway of the trunk and limbs

　　C. The fasciculus gracilis

　　D. The fasciculus cuneatus

11. Conduction of the tactile and pressure sensation from the head and face to the brainstem is (　　).

　　A. spinal nuclei of trigeminal nerve

　　B. midbrain nuclei of trigeminal nerve

　　C. pontine nuclei of trigeminal nerve

　　D. nucleus of solitary tract

12. About the superficial sensory pathway of the trunk and limbs, which of the following statements is **wrong**? (　　)

　　A. The third neurons are located in ventroposterolateral nucleus of thalamus.

　　B. Lateral spinothalamic tract conduct the rude tactile and pressure sensation.

　　C. The fibers which come from second neurons intersect at spinal cord.

　　D. Central radiation of thalamus conduct pain and thermal sensation, the rude tactile and pressure sensation.

13. Ventroposteromedial nucleus of thalamus receives (　　).

　　A. medial lemniscus

    B. lateral lemniscus

    C. trigeminal lemniscus

    D. spinothalamic tract

14. The first neurons of visual pathway are (   ).

    A. rod and cone cells

    B. bipolar cells

    C. ganglion cells

    D. lateral geniculate body

15. The injury of left optic tract may cause (   ).

    A. blindness of left eye

    B. temporal hemianopia of right eye, nasal hemianopia of left eye

    C. temporal hemianopia of both eyes

    D. temporal hemianopia of left eye, nasal hemianopia of right eye

16. The injury of central part of optic chiasma may cause (   ).

    A. nasal hemianopia of both eyes

    B. nasal hemianopia of left eye

    C. temporal hemianopia of both eyes

    D. blindness of both eyes

17. The injury of left oculomotor nerve may cause (   ).

    A. the right eye disappears directly to the pupillary light reflex

    B. the left eye disappears indirectly to the pupillary light reflex

    C. the direct pupillary light reflex of left eye is normal

    D. the right eye disappears indirectly to the pupillary light reflex

18. About the fasciculus gracilis and the fasciculus cuneatus, which of the following statements is true? (   )

    A. It is located in the posterior funiculus of the spinal cord.

    B. It is located in the lateral funiculus of the spinal cord.

    C. It is located in the anterior funiculus of the spinal cord.

    D. It is located in brain stem.

19. The structure independent of acoustic pathway is (   ).

    A. cochlear nucleus

    B. lateral geniculate body

    C. lateral lemniscus

    D. transverse temporal gyrus

20. The position of the left joint can **not** be determined when the eyes are closed, this may be caused by the damage of (   ).

    A. right medial lemniscus

    B. right lateral lemniscus

    C. right trigeminal lemniscus

    D. left spinothalamic tract

21. In contralateral somatosensory disorder, structures that may be damaged do **not** include (   ).

    A. postcentral gyrus

    B. central radiation of thalamus

    C. the posterior limb of the internal capsule

    D. lateral lemniscus

22. About the pyramidal system, which statement is **wrong**? (   )

    A. It contains the corticospinal tract.

    B. It contains the corticonuclear tract.

    C. It contains three order neurons.

    D. The cell body of superior motor neurons are located in the anterior central gyrus and paracentric lobules.

23. What is independent of the injuries of superior motor neurons? (   )

    A. Spastic paralysis

    B. Increased muscular tension

    C. Tendon hyperreflexia

    D. Negative pathological reflex

24. The fibers of corticonuclear tract come from (   ).

    A. the upper and middle parts of the postcentral gyrus, and the posterior part of the paracentral lobule

    B. the inferior part of the postcentral gyrus

    C. the upper and middle parts of the precentral gyrus, and the anterior part of the paracentral lobule

    D. the inferior part of the precentral gyrus

25. The injury of corticospinal tract on one side of spinal cord leads to (   ).

    A. ipsilateral paralysis and increased muscular tension

    B. the ipsilateral paralysis and tendon reflex disappeared

    C. the contralateral limb paralysis and tendon reflex disappeared

    D. the contralateral limb paralysis and decreased muscular tension

26. The corticospinal tract mainly innervates the movement of skeletal muscle of (   ).

    A. ipsilateral upper and lower limb

    B. contralateral upper and lower limb

    C. ipsilateral trunk and limbs

    D. both trunk and limbs

27. The nucleus that receives only the fibers of the contralateral corticonuclear tract is (   ).

    A. motor nucleus of trigeminal nerve

    B. nucleus of trochlear nerve

    C. nucleus of hypoglossal nerve

    D. nucleus of abducent nerve

28. Which of the following structures may cause paralysis of the contralateral lingual muscle after injury? (　　)

    A. Rubrospinal tract

    B. Corticonuclear tract

    C. Corticospinal tract

    D. Posterior limb of internal capsule

29. Injury of the left corticonuclear tract will result in the paralysis of the (　　).

    A. right facial muscles below the palpebral fissure

    B. right facial muscle above the palpebral fissure

    C. left facial muscles below the palpebral fissure

    D. left facial muscles above the palpebral fissure

30. Which of the following structures dominates the lower facial muscle? (　　)

    A. Ipsilateral corticonuclear tract

    B. Contralateral corticonuclear tract

    C. Ipsilateral corticospinal tract

    D. Contralateral corticospinal tract

II. Double choices (Choose the two best answers among the following choices, and write down the corresponding letters in bracket)

1. Which ones of the following structures are associated with superficial sensory pathway of trunk and limbs? (　　)

    A. Spinal ganglion

    B. Medial lemniscus

    C. Ventroposteromedial nucleus of thalamus

    D. Central radiation of thalamus

    E. Inferior part of postcentral gyrus

2. Which ones of the following pathways are associated with central radiation of thalamus? (　　)

    A. Rubrospinal tract

    B. Medial lemniscus

    C. Spinothalamic tract

    D. Corticonuclear tract

    E. Corticospinal tract

3. Neurons that do **not** belong to the visual pathway are (　　).

    A. medial geniculate body

    B. rod and cone cells

C. lateral geniculate body

D. bipolar cells

E. ganglion cells

4. The sensory pathways whose the third order neuron is in the ventroposterolateral nucleus of the thalamus are (   ).

A. visual pathway

B. the superficial sensory pathway of trunk and limbs

C. the superficial sensory pathway of head and face

D. acoustic pathway

E. the deep sensory pathway of trunk and limbs

5. About the deep sensory pathway of trunk and limbs, which ones of the following statements are true? (   )

A. Second neurons are gracile and cuneate nuclei.

B. Most of the fibers cross through the anterior white commissure to the contralateral anterolateral cord and run upward.

C. Third neurons are ventroposterolateral nucleus.

D. Pass through anterior limb of internal capsule.

E. The fibers crossing in spinal cord.

6. The structures which pass through posterior limb of internal capsule are (   ).

A. central thalamic radiation

B. corticospinal tract

C. anterior thalamic radiation

D. frontopontine tract

E. corticonuclear tract

7. About the pyramidal system, which ones of the following statements are **wrong**? (   )

A. Pathological reflex is positive after injury.

B. It is divided into corticospinal tract and corticonuclear tract.

C. Lateral corticospinal tract controls ipsilateral muscles of limbs.

D. The cell bodies of the superior motor neurons are located in the postcentral gyrus and the posterior part paracentral lobule.

E. The fibers crossing are all in the medulla oblongata.

8. Corticospinal tract injury can lead to (   ).

A. spastic paralysis

B. muscle atrophy

C. superficial hyperreflexia

D. deep hyporeflexia

E. pathological reflex positive

9. Corticonuclear tract injury can lead to (   ).

    A. the contralateral expression muscle is paralysis above the eye fissure

    B. contralateral masticatory is paralysis

    C. the contralateral expression muscle is paralysis below the eye fissure

    D. contralateral ophthalmoplegia

    E. contralateral lingual paralysis

10. The structures associated with trigeminal lemniscus are (　　).

    A. trigeminal ganglion

    B. nucleus of facial nerve

    C. ventroposteromedial nucleus of thalamus

    D. inferior part of precentral gyrus

    E. anterior limb of internal capsule

Ⅲ. Fill the blanks (Fill the most appropriate words in the blanks)

1. The pyramidal system includes the _____ and the _____.

2. The sensory pathways of the first neurons in the spinal ganglia are _____ and _____.

3. The superficial sensory pathway of the trunk and limbs is composed of three grade neurons. First neurons are _____, second neurons are _____, third neurons are _____.

4. The deep sensory pathway of the trunk and limbs is composed of three grade neurons. First neurons are _____, second neurons are _____, third neurons are _____.

5. Central radiation of thalamus is the continuation of _____, _____, and _____.

6. The visual pathway is composed of three grade neurons. First neurons are _____, second neurons are _____, third neurons are _____.

7. Optic tract contains the _____ and _____.

8. The fibers ending in the ventroposteromedial nucleus of thalamus are called _____, and they pass though _____, project into _____.

9. The fibers which come from the ventroposterolateral nucleus of thalamus are called _____, pass though _____, projected into _____ and _____.

10. The pathway passing through the genu of internal capsule is called _____.

11. The cell bodies of the superior motor neurons of corticospinal tract are located in _____ and _____.

12. The pathways, which pass through posterior limb of internal capsule, are _____, _____, _____ and _____.

13. The superficial sensory pathway of head and face is composed of three grade neurons. First neurons are _____, second neurons are _____, and _____.

14. The axons of the upper motor neurons of pyramidal system form _____ and

_____.

15. The sensory pathway that crosses in the spinal cord is _____.

IV. Answer questions briefly

1. Please describe the visual pathway.
2. Please describe the pupillary reflexes.
3. Please describe the superficial sensory pathway of face and head.
4. Please describe the upper motor neurons.
5. Please describe the formation and function of extrapyramidal system.

V. Answer questions in detail

1. Please describe the superficial sensory pathway of trunk and limbs.
2. Please describe the deep sensory pathway of trunk and limbs.
3. Please describe the corticospinal tract pathway.

VI. Problems in life

1. Does the most intelligent people have the largest brain?
2. What do our earliest memories recall?

Chapter 22   The Meninges and Blood Vessels and the Cerebrospinal Fluid

Ⅰ. **Single choice（Choose the best answer among the following four choices, and write down the corresponding letter in bracket）**

1. The artery arising from the basilar artery is （　　）.
    A. anterior cerebral artery
    B. middle cerebral artery
    C. posterior cerebral artery
    D. ophthalmic artery

2. Which of the following artery is **not** involved in the formation of the cerebral arterial circle of Willis? （　　）
    A. Anterior cerebral artery
    B. Middle cerebral artery
    C. Posterior cerebral artery
    D. Posterior communicating artery

3. Which of the following space formed by the meninges of spinal cord contains lymphatic vessels and venous plexuses? （　　）
    A. Epidural space
    B. Subarachnoid space
    C. Subdural space
    D. Terminal cistern

4. Which of the following space is filled by the cerebrospinal fluid? （　　）
    A. Subdural space
    B. Subarachnoid space
    C. Vertebral canal
    D. Epidural space

5. The total volume of cerebrospinal fluid in adults is around （　　）.
    A. 500 mL
    B. 1000 mL
    C. 50 mL
    D. 150 mL

6. The cerebrospinal fluid is mainly produced by （　　）.
    A. cerebral arachnoid mater
    B. cerebral pia mater
    C. choroid plexuses of cerebral ventricles

D. lymphatic vessels

7. The fracture of skull usually leads to (   ).

A. subdural hematoma

B. subarachnoid hemorrhage

C. epidural hematoma

D. lateral ventricular hemorrhage

8. Which of the following sinuses of dura mater may be injured by the fracture of parietal bone? (   )

A. Superior sagittal sinus

B. Cavernous sinus

C. Transverse sinus

D. Inferior sagittal sinus

9. The somatic motor area is mainly supplied by (   ).

A. cortical branches of anterior cerebral artery

B. central branches of anterior cerebral artery

C. cortical branches of middle cerebral artery

D. central branches of middle cerebral artery

10. The somatic sensory area is mainly supplied by (   ).

A. cortical branches of anterior cerebral artery

B. central branches of anterior cerebral artery

C. cortical branches of middle cerebral artery

D. central branches of middle cerebral artery

11. Which of the following arteries runs through the cavernous sinus? (   )

A. Middle cerebral artery

B. Vertebral artery

C. Posterior cerebral artery

D. Internal carotid artery

12. The language areas is mainly supplied by (   ).

A. anterior choroid artery

B. posterior cerebral artery

C. anterior cerebral artery

D. middle cerebral artery

13. Which of the following arteries supplies the internal capsule? (   )

A. Cortical branches of anterior cerebral artery

B. Central branches of anterior cerebral artery

C. Cortical branches of posterior cerebral artery

D. Central branches of posterior cerebral artery

14. The septa that separates the cerebellum from cerebrum is (   ).

A. cerebral falx

    B. cerebellar falx

    C. tentorium of cerebellum

    D. diaphragm sellae

15. Which of the following statements about the sinus of dura mater is **wrong**? (　　)

    A. The cerebral veins are drained into the sinus.

    B. The wall of the sinus lacks of smooth muscles.

    C. The sigmoid sinus drains the transverse sinus into the internal jugular vein.

    D. The oculomotor nerve runs through the internal wall of cavernous sinus.

16. Which of the following subarachnoid cistern is the largest? (　　)

    A. Pontine cistern

    B. Interpeduncular cistern

    C. Chiasmatic cistern

    D. Cerebellomedullary cistern

17. Which of the following arteriesis particularly susceptible to damage from the hypertension? (　　)

    A. Cortical branches of anterior cerebral artery

    B. Central branches of anterior cerebral artery

    C. Cortical branches of middle cerebral artery

    D. Central branches of middle cerebral artery

18. The lenticulostriate arteries arise from (　　).

    A. anterior artery

    B. posterior communicating artery

    C. anterior communicating artery

    D. middle cerebral artery

19. About tentorialincisure, which of the following statement is **wrong**? (　　)

    A. The incisure is the free anterior border of the cerebellar tentorium.

    B. The parahippocampal gyrus and uncus are located above the incisure.

    C. The pons is surrounded by the hole between the incisure and dorsum sellae.

    D. Intracranial hypertension can lead to tentorial hernia, thus pressing the oculomotor nerve.

20. The cavernous sinus drains the blood from the following veins, **except** (　　).

    A. inferior cerebral veins

    B. superficial middle cerebral veins

    C. ophthalmic vein

    D. internal cerebral vein

21. About cavernous sinus, which of the following statement is **incorrect**? (　　)

    A. It is located on each side of the sella turcica.

    B. Vertebral artery runs through its internal wall.

    C. Oculomotor nerve passes through its lateral wall.

D. Ophthalmic vein drains into it.

22. Which of the following artery is **not** a branch of internal carotid artery? (　　)

A. Anterior cerebral artery

B. Middle cerebral artery

C. Posterior communicating artery

D. Posterior cerebral artery

23. Which of the following artery is **not** a branch of vertebral artery? (　　)

A. Anterior spinal artery

B. Posterior inferior cerebellar artery

C. Posterior spinal artery

D. Posterior communicating artery

24. The spinal cord is supplied by the following arteries, **except** (　　).

A. posterior communicating artery

B. anterior spinal artery

C. posterior spinal artery

D. lumbar arteries

25. About the cerebral arterial circle, which of the following statement is correct?
(　　)

A. Middle cerebral artery joins to form the circle.

B. It is located below the hypophysis.

C. It encircles the optic chiasma, the tuber cinereum and the mammillary bodies.

D. The circle communicates the left vertebral artery with right one.

26. Which of the following structure is **not** a component of the blood-brain barrier?
(　　)

A. Capillary endothelium

B. Homogenous basement membrane

C. Choroids plexus

D. Neuroglial membrane formed by the processes of the astrocytes

27. Which of the following area is devoid of a blood-brain barrier? (　　)

A. Cerebellar hemispheres

B. Dorsal thalamus

C. Hippocampus

D. Pituitary gland

28. Which of the following septa divides the intracranial cavity into supratentorial and
infratentorial parts? (　　)

A. Cerebral falx

B. Diaphragm sellae

C. Cerebellar falx

D. Tentorium of cerebellum

29. In the vertebral canal, which of the following space is usually applicable for block anesthesia? (   )

    A. Epidural space

    B. Subarachnoid space

    C. Subdural space

    D. Terminal cistern

30. About the meninges of brain and spinal cord, which of the following is **incorrect**? (   )

    A. From outside to inside, there are dura mater, arachnoid and pia mater.

    B. Spinal and cerebral dura maters are continuous at the foramen magnum.

    C. Arachnoid mater is rich in blood vessels.

    D. Spinal dura mater is continuous with the meninges of spinal nerves.

II. Double choices (Choose the two best answers among the following choices, and write down the corresponding letters in bracket)

1. Which ones of the following structures run through the internal wall of cavernous sinus? (   )

    A. Internal carotid artery

    B. Middle cerebral artery

    C. Posterior cerebral artery

    D. Abducent nerve

    E. Oculomotor nerve

2. Which ones of the following arteries are **not** the components of the cerebral arterial circle of Willis? (   )

    A. Anterior cerebral artery

    B. Middle cerebral artery

    C. Posterior cerebral artery

    D. Internal carotid artery

    E. Anterior choroid artery

3. The arteries arising from the internal carotid artery are (   ).

    A. anterior cerebral artery

    B. posterior communicating artery

    C. posterior cerebral artery

    D. basilar artery

    E. labyrinthine artery

4. Which ones of the following veins are drained by the cavernous sinus? (   )

    A. Inferior cerebral veins

    B. Internal jugular vein

    C. Ophthalmic vein

D. Internal cerebral vein

E. Great cerebral vein

5. About the meninges of brain and spinal cord, which ones of the following statement are **incorrect**? (   )

A. From outside to inside, there are dura mater, arachnoid and pia mater.

B. Spinal and cerebral dura maters are continuous at the foramen magnum.

C. Arachnoid mater is rich in blood vessels.

D. Spinal dura mater is continuous with the meninges of spinal nerves at intervertebral foramina.

E. Denticulate ligament is formed by the spinal dura mater.

6. The confluence of sinus is a direct confluence of (   ).

A. sigmoid sinus

B. cavernous sinus

C. inferior sagittal sinus

D. straight sinus

E. superior sagittal sinus

7. Which of the following arteries do **not** supply the internal capsule? (   )

A. Posterior cerebral artery

B. Anterior cerebral artery

C. Middle cerebral artery

D. Anterior choroid artery

E. Vertebral artery

8. The arteries arising from the basilar artery are (   ).

A. anterior cerebral artery

B. middle cerebral artery

C. posterior cerebral artery

D. ophthalmic artery

E. superior cerebellar artery

9. About lenticulostriate arteries, which ones of the following statements are **incorrect**?

(   )

A. They arise from anterior cerebral artery.

B. They supply the somatic motor, somatic sensory and language areas.

C. The wall of the arteries is thinner.

D. They travel directly upward from the stem.

E. The regions they supply have significant collateral blood supplement.

10. About the cerebral spinal fluid (CSF), which ones of the following statements are **incorrect**? (   )

A. CSF is clear, colorless fluid in the brain and spinal cord.

B. CSF is produced by the choroid plexuses of the ventricles of the brain.

C. CSF is absorbed in the arachnoid granulations.

D. CSF occupies the subdural space, ventricular system as well as the central canal of the spinal cord.

E. CSF moves multidirectionally in the ventricles of brain.

III. Fill the blanks (Fill the most appropriate words in the blanks)

1. From outside to inside, the three layers of membranes of the brain are _____, _____ and _____.

2. The CSF is absorbed in the _____.

3. _____ divides the intracranial cavity into supratentorial and infratentorial parts.

4. The brain barriers are composed of _____, _____ and _____.

5. _____ and _____ run through the internal wall of cavernous sinus.

6. The cerebral spinal fluid in the lateral ventricle passes through _____ to the third ventricle, then through the _____ to the fourth ventricle.

7. The gap between the two layers of cerebral dura mater is called _____.

8. The brain receives the blood from the _____ and _____.

9. The dura mater that partially separates the cerebellar hemispheres is _____, and partially separates the cerebellum from cerebrum is _____.

10. The free anterior border of the cerebellar tentorium is called _____.

11. The cerebral branches of internal carotid artery include _____, _____, _____ and _____.

12. The circle of Willis is composed of the following arteries: _____, _____, _____, _____, _____ and _____.

13. All arteries forming the cerebral arterial circle give off two types of branches. They are _____ branches and _____ branches.

14. The blood-brain barrier is formed by _____, _____, and _____.

15. In the telencephalon, _____ arteries are particularly susceptible to damage from hypertension.

IV. Answer questions briefly

1. Please describe the course of the internal carotid artery.

2. Please describe the origins of arteries that forming the circle of Willis.

3. Please describe the circulation of cerebrospinal fluid.

4. Please describe the main reflections formed by the cerebral dura mater.

5. Please describe the characteristics of sinuses of dura mater and clinical relevance.

6. Please describe the structures that run through the cavernous sinus.

7. Please describe the blood supply of the spinal cord.

V. Answer questions in detail

1. Please describe the cerebral branches of internal carotid artery and their functions.

2. Please describe the source, location and circulation of cerebrospinal fluid.

3. Please describe the meninges of spinal cord and main clinical relevances.

Chapter 23　The Spinal Nerves

Ⅰ. **Single choice（Choose the best answer among the following four choices, and write down the corresponding letter in bracket）**

1. Which nerve belongs to branches of cervical plexus? (　　)
   A. Thoracodorsal nerve
   B. Phrenic nerve
   C. Axillary nerve
   D. Facial nerve

2. Which nerve belongs to the branches of posterior cord of the brachial plexus? (　　)
   A. Axillary nerve
   B. Median nerve
   C. Dorsal scapular nerve
   D. Musculocutaneous nerve

3. Which nerve belongs to the branches of medial cord of the brachial plexus? (　　)
   A. Axillary nerve
   B. Long thoracic nerve
   C. Ulnar nerve
   D. Musculocutaneous nerve

4. Which nerve belongs to the branches of lateral cord of the brachial plexus? (　　)
   A. Dorsal scapular nerve
   B. Radial nerve
   C. Thoracodorsal nerve
   D. Musculocutaneous nerve

5. Which nerve is given off by the lumbar plexus? (　　)
   A. Sciatic nerve
   B. Pudendal nerve
   C. Posterior femoral cutaneous nerve
   D. Obturator nerve

6. Which nerve is **not** given off by the lumbar plexus? (　　)
   A. Ilioinguinal nerve
   B. Genitofemoral nerve
   C. Posterior femoral cutaneous nerve
   D. Obturator nerve

7. Which nerve is given off by the sacral plexus? (　　)
   A. Ilioinguinal nerve

   B. Genitofemoral nerve

   C. Posterior femoral cutaneous nerve

   D. Lateral femoral cutaneous nerve

8. Which nerve is **not** given off by the sacral plexus? (   )

   A. Sciatic nerve

   B. Lateral femoral cutaneous nerve

   C. Superior gluteal nerve

   D. Pudendal nerve

9. Which of the following statements about the spinal nerve is **not** true? (   )

   A. The spinal ganglia contain pseudounipolar neurons.

   B. The anterior branch of the spinal nerve contains sensory and motor fibers.

   C. The posterior branch of the spinal nerve only contains sensory fibers.

   D. The communicating branches connect with the sympathetic trunk.

10. Which of the following statements about the phrenic nerve is **not** true? (   )

   A. It is one of the muscular branches of the cervical plexus.

   B. It is the longest branch of the cervical plexus.

   C. It innervates the diaphragm.

   D. The fibers of the left phrenic nerve are also distributed to the liver, gallbladder
      and the bile duct system.

11. Which of the following statements about the superficial branches of cervical plexus
    is true? (   )

   A. They emerge near the middle of the posterior border of the sternocleidomastoid.

   B. They only contain somatic motor fibers.

   C. They emerge near the middle of the anterior border of the sternocleidomastoid.

   D. Great occipital nerve is one of the superficial branches of cervical plexus.

12. Which of the following statements about the cervical plexus is true? (   )

   A. It is formed by the first three cervical nerves.

   B. It is covered by the sternocleidomastoid.

   C. It is covered by the scalenus medius.

   D. Its branches are only distributed to the skin of neck.

13. Which nerve belongs to the branches of brachial plexus above the clavicle? (   )

   A. Thoracodorsal nerve

   B. Long thoracic nerve

   C. Medial pectoral nerve

   D. Lateral pectoral nerve

14. Which of the following statements about the ulnar nerve is **not** true? (   )

   A. It arises from the medial cord of the brachial plexus.

   B. It has no branch in the arm.

   C. Its cutaneous branches are distributed to the skin of ulnar side of the forearm.

    D. It innervates the hypothenar muscles.

15. Which nerve after injury results in "ape-like" hand? (　　)

    A. Axillary nerve

    B. Ulnar nerve

    C. Median nerve

    D. Radial nerve

16. Which nerve after injury results in "wristdrop"? (　　)

    A. Median nerve

    B. Ulnar nerve

    C. Axillary nerve

    D. Radial nerve

17. Which of the following statements about the radial nerve is **not** true? (　　)

    A. It arises from the posterior cord of the brachial plexus.

    B. It innervates the brachioradialis.

    C. Its cutaneous branches are distributed to the skin of posterior aspect of the arm.

    D. It innervates the deltoid.

18. Which of the following statements about the median nerve is **not** true? (　　)

    A. It belongs to branches of the medial cord of the brachial plexus.

    B. It has no branch in the arm.

    C. It innervates the first and second lumbrical muscles.

    D. It innervates the thenar muscles except for the adductor pollicis.

19. Which nerve after injury results in "clawhand"? (　　)

    A. Median nerve

    B. Ulnar nerve

    C. Radial nerve

    D. Axillary nerve

20. Which of the following statements about the axillary nerve is **not** true? (　　)

    A. It arises from the posterior cord of the brachial plexus.

    B. It has no branch in the arm.

    C. It innervates the deltoid.

    D. It passes through the quadrangular space.

21. About the axillary nerve, which of the following statements is true? (　　)

    A. It arises from the lateral cord of the brachial plexus.

    B. It has no branch in the arm.

    C. It innervates the deltoid.

    D. It passes through the triangular space.

22. Which of the following statements about the thoracic nerves is true? (　　)

    A. The anterior branches of the thoracic nerves form 12 pairs of intercostal nerves.

    B. The intercostal nerve accompanies the posterior intercostal vessels.

    C. The anterior cutaneous branches of the second thoracic nerve are distributed to the skin of the thoracic wall at the level of nipple.

    D. The anterior cutaneous branches of the thoracic nerves are only distributed to the skin of the thoracic wall.

23. Which nerve innervates sartorius? (   )

    A. Obturator nerve

    B. Ilioinguinal nerve

    C. Genitofemoral nerve

    D. Femoral nerve

24. Which nerve, when injured, would result in impaired adduction of the thigh? (   )

    A. Obturator nerve

    B. Ilioinguinal nerve

    C. Genitofemoral nerve

    D. Femoral nerve

25. Which of the following statements about the femoral nerve is true? (   )

    A. It descends beneath the inguinal ligament into femoral triangle.

    B. It only controls the sensation on the skin of the anterior aspect of thigh.

    C. It innervates the adductor longus.

    D. It controls the sensation of the most skin of the dorsum of foot.

26. Which of the following statements about the femoral nerve is **not** true? (   )

    A. It descends beneath the inguinal ligament into femoral triangle.

    B. It innervates the quadriceps femoris.

    C. One of its cutaneous nerves is the saphenous nerve.

    D. It innervates the gracilis.

27. Which of the following statements about the obturator nerve is true? (   )

    A. It emerges from the lateral border of the psoas major.

    B. It innervates most medial muscles of the thigh.

    C. It innervates the semitendinosus.

    D. It controls the sensation on the skin of the anterior aspect of the thigh.

28. Which of the following statements about the obturator nerve is **not** true? (   )

    A. It emerges from the medial border of the psoas major.

    B. It innervates most medial muscles of the thigh.

    C. It controls the sensation on the skin of the medial aspect of the leg and foot.

    D. It controls the sensation on the skin of the medial aspect of the thigh.

29. Which of the following statements about the sacral plexus is true? (   )

    A. It is formed by the sacral and coccygeal nerves.

    B. It is located in the pelvis.

    C. It is formed by posterior branches of the sacral and coccygeal nerves.

  D. Its cutaneous branches are distributed throughout the skin of the foot.

 30. Which of the following statements about the sciatic nerve is **not** true? ( )

  A. It is the largest nerve in the body.

  B. Its terminal branches are the tibial nerve and the peroneal nerve.

  C. It innervates all muscles of the leg and foot.

  D. It controls the sensation on the skin of theposterior aspect of the leg.

 31. Which of the following statements about the sciatic nerve is true? ( )

  A. It is the largest nerve in the body.

  B. Its terminal branches are the tibial nerve and the peroneal nerve.

  C. It innervates all muscles of the thigh.

  D. Its cutaneous branches are distributed throughout the skin of the foot.

 32. Which of the following does **not** leave the pelvis through the infrapiriform foramen?
  ( )

  A. Inferior gluteal nerve

  B. Superior gluteal nerve

  C. Posterior femoral cutaneous nerve

  D. Pudendal nerve

 33. Which of the following statements about the tibial nerve is true? ( )

  A. It is one of the terminal branches of the sciatic nerve.

  B. It innervates the muscles of the lateral compartment of the leg.

  C. It innervates the muscles of the anterior compartment of the leg.

  D. It gives off the lateral sural cutaneous nerve.

 34. Which of the following statements about the common peroneal nerve is **not** true?
  ( )

  A. It is one of the terminal branches of the sciatic nerve.

  B. It innervates the muscles of the lateral compartment of the leg.

  C. It innervates the muscles of the anterior compartment of the leg.

  D. It gives off the medial sural cutaneous nerve.

 35. Which of the following statements about the deep peroneal nerve is true? ( )

  A. It has no cutaneous branch on the skin of the dorsum of the foot.

  B. It innervates the muscles of the anterior compartment of the leg.

  C. It gives off the lateral sural cutaneous nerve.

  D. It gives off the medial sural cutaneous nerve.

II. Double choices(Choose the two best answers among the following choices, and write down the corresponding letters in bracket)

 1. Which nerves control the sensation on the skin of the anterior and medial aspect of the thigh? ( )

  A. Iliohypogastric nerve

    B. Obturator nerve

    C. Femoral nerve

    D. Ilioinguinal nerve

    E. Saphenous nerve

2. Which nerves leave the pelvis through the infrapiriform foramen? (   )

    A. Inferior gluteal nerve

    B. Genitofemoral nerve

    C. Lateral femoral cutaneous nerve

    D. Superior gluteal nerve

    E. Sciatic nerve

3. Which nerves give off the branches to form the sural nerve? (   )

    A. Tibial nerve

    B. Superficial peroneal nerve

    C. Deep peroneal nerve

    D. Common peroneal nerve

    E. Femoral nerve

4. Which ones of the following contain both sensory and motor fibers? (   )

    A. Anterior root of the spinal nerve

    B. Posterior root of the spinal nerve

    C. Anterior branch of the spinal nerve

    D. Posterior branch of the spinal nerve

    E. Communicating branches of the spinal nerve

5. Which ones of the following belong to the cutaneous branches of the cervical plexus?

    (   )

    A. Lesser occipital nerve

    B. Greater occipital nerve

    C. Suprascapular nerve

    D. Phrenic nerve

    E. Supraclavicular nerve

6. Which ones of the following are innervated by the ulnar nerve? (   )

    A. The first and second lumbricales

    B. Biceps brachii

    C. Interosseous muscles

    D. Flexor digitorum superficialis

    E. Hypothenar muscles

7. Which nerves have **no** branches in the arm? (   )

    A. Ulnar nerve

    B. Radial nerve

    C. Median nerve

    D. Axillary nerve

    E. Musculocutaneous nerve

8. Which nerves control the sensation of the palmar skin? (　　)

    A. Radial nerve

    B. Ulnar nerve

    C. Axillary nerve

    D. Musculocutaneous nerve

    E. Median nerve

9. Which nerves do **not** control the sensation of the skin of the dorsum of the hand?
（　　）

    A. Radial nerve

    B. Axillary nerve

    C. Median nerve

    D. Musculocutaneous nerve

    E. Ulnar nerve

10. Which ones of the following are innervated by the radial nerve? (　　)

    A. Pronator teres

    B. Interosseous muscles

    C. Pronator quadratus

    D. Brachioradialis

    E. Triceps brachii

11. Which ones of the following are innervated by the femoral nerve? (　　)

    A. Sartorius

    B. Gracilis

    C. Biceps femoris

    D. Quadriceps femoris

    E. Tensor fasciae latae

12. Which ones of the following are innervated by the deep peroneal nerve? (　　)

    A. Tibialis anterior

    B. Extensor halluces longus

    C. Tibialis posterior

    D. Flexor digitorum longus

    E. Soleus

13. Which ones of the following are innervated by the tibial nerve? (　　)

    A. Tibialis anterior

    B. Extensor digitorum longus

    C. Tibialis posterior

    D. Flexor halluces longus

    E. Peroneus longus

14. Which ones of the following are given off by the posterior cord of the brachial plexus? (   )
    A. Lateral pectoral nerve
    B. Median nerve
    C. Musculocutaneous nerve
    D. Axillary nerve
    E. Radial nerve
15. Which nerves, when injured, cause "foot-drop" or "talipes equinovarus"? (   )
    A. Tibial nerve
    B. Superficial peroneal nerve
    C. Deep peroneal nerve
    D. Femoral nerve
    E. Sural nerve

Ⅲ. Fill the blanks (Fill the most appropriate words in the blanks)

1. The four types of fibers in the spinal nerves are _____ , _____ , _____ and _____ .
2. After leaving the intervertebral foramen, each spinal nerve is divided into _____ , _____ , _____ , and _____ branches.
3. The cutaneous branches of cervical plexus are _____ , _____ , _____ , and _____ .
4. The brachial plexus is formed by the anterior branches of _____ .
5. The muscles of the anterior group in the arm include _____ , _____ and _____ , which are innervated by _____ nerve.
6. The muscles of the anterior group in the forearm are innervated by _____ , _____ and _____ nerves.
7. The sensation of the skin of the palmar is controlled by _____ and _____ nerves.
8. The anterior branches of the second thoracic nerve are distributed at the _____ level, the anterior branches of the tenth thoracic nerve are distributed at the _____ level.
9. Besides the sciatic nerve, _____ , _____ and _____ nerves also pass through the infrapiriform foramen.
10. The sensation of the skin of the sole is controlled by _____ nerve.
11. The muscles of the posterior group in the thigh are _____ and _____ , and they are innervated by _____ nerve.
12. The branches of the lumbar plexus, which emerge from the lateral border of the psoas major, are _____ , _____ , _____ , and _____ nerves.
13. The lumbosacral trunk is formed by _____ and _____ .

14. The sural nerve is formed by _____ given off by _____ , and _____ given off by _____ .

15. The muscles of the lateral group in the leg are _____ and _____ ; they are innervated by _____ nerve.

IV. Answer questions briefly

1. Please briefly describe the name and formation of four plexuses.
2. Please briefly describe the name and distribution of the 4 branches of spinal nerve.
3. Please describe the superficial branches and distribution of the cervical plexus.
4. Please describe the name and innervation nerves of the muscles in arm.
5. Please describe the name and innervation nerves of the muscles in thigh.
6. Please briefly describe the symptoms of injury of the axillary nerve and analysis the cause.
7. Please briefly describe the symptoms of injury of the femoral nerve and analysis the cause.
8. Please describe the name and innervation nerves of the muscles in leg.

V. Answer questions in detail

1. Please describe the distribution characteristics of the anterior branches of the 12 pairs of thoracic nerves.
2. Please describe the muscles and skin area controlled by sciatic nerve and its terminal branches.

VI. Problems in life

1. What is spinal tap?
2. What is the "funny bone"?
3. Why does your foot sometimes "fall asleep"?

Chapter 24   The Cranial Nerves

I. **Single choice (Choose the best answer among the following four choices, and write down the corresponding letter in bracket)**

1. The nerve containing the general visceral motor fibers is (   ).
   A. oculomotor nerve
   B. trigeminal nerve
   C. abducent nerve
   D. hypoglossal nerve

2. Which of the following controls the secretion of lacrimal gland? (   )
   A. Trigeminal nerve
   B. Oculomotor nerve
   C. Trochlear nerve
   D. Facial nerve

3. Which of the following supplies the expression muscles? (   )
   A. Facial nerve
   B. Trigeminal nerve
   C. Infraobital nerve
   D. Frontal nerve

4. Which of the following is a special somatic sensory nerve? (   )
   A. Olfactory nerve
   B. Oculomotor nerve
   C. Trochlear nerve
   D. Optic nerve

5. Which nerve contains visceral sensory fibers? (   )
   A. Trigeminal nerve
   B. Oculomotor nerve
   C. Vagus nerve
   D. Abducent nerve

6. Which of the following is a pure motor nerve? (   )
   A. Trigeminal nerve
   B. Oculomotor nerve
   C. Facial nerve
   D. Glossopharyngeal nerve

7. Which of the following regulates the size of the pupil? (   )
   A. Optic nerve

    B. Trochlear nerve

    C. Oculomotor nerve

    D. Ophthalmic nerve

8. Which of the following innervates the levator palpebrae superioris? (　　)

    A. Trochlear nerve

    B. Oculomotor nerve

    C. Abducent nerve

    D. Frontal nerve

9. Which of the following statements about oculomotor nerve is **not** true? (　　)

    A. It passes through the superior orbital fissure.

    B. It enters into the orbit through the medial wall of the cavernous sinus.

    C. It innervates most of the extraocular muscles.

    D. It contains two types of motor fibers.

10. Which of the following statements about optic nerve is **not** true? (　　)

    A. It is a special visceral sensory nerve.

    B. It passes through the optic canal.

    C. It originates from the ganglionic cells of the retina.

    D. It is enclosed in three layers of the coverings.

11. The trochlear nerve innervates (　　).

    A. rectus medialis

    B. obliquus superior

    C. rectus lateralis

    D. obliquus inferior

12. Which of the following statements about trochlear nerve is **not** true? (　　)

    A. It is a special visceral motor nerve.

    B. It passes through the superior orbital fissure.

    C. It innervates the superior obliquus.

    D. It enters into the orbit through the lateral wall of the cavernous sinus.

13. Two types of fibers in the trigeminal nerve are (　　)

    A. the special visceral motorand general visceral sensory fibers

    B. the general visceral sensory and general somatic motor fibers

    C. the special visceral sensory and general visceral motor fibers

    D. the general somatic sensory and the special visceral motor fibers

14. The trigeminal nerve innervates (　　)

    A. posterior belly of digastric muscle

    B. masseter

    C. platysma

    D. stylohyoid

15. The following branches arise in the facial canal **except** (　　)

A.　the lesser petrosal nerve

B.　the greater petrosal nerve

C.　the chorda tympani nerve

D.　the stapedius branch of the facial nerve

16.　Which of the following is **not** included in the facial nerve? (　　)

A.　General somatic sensory fibers

B.　General visceral sensory fibers

C.　General visceral motor fibers

D.　Special visceral motor fibers

17.　The fibers innervating the expression muscles belong to (　　)

A.　the special visceral motor fibers

B.　the general visceral motor fibers

C.　the general somatic motor fibers

D.　the special somatic sensory fibers

18.　The following ganglia belong to the parasympathetic ganglia **except** (　　)

A.　otic ganglion

B.　geniculate ganglion

C.　submandibular ganglion

D.　ciliary ganglion

19.　Which of the following statements about facial nerve is **not** true? (　　)

A.　It passes through the stylomastoid foramen.

B.　It contains 4 types of fibers.

C.　It controls the secretion of parotid gland.

D.　It controls taste sense of the anterior 2/3 of the tongue.

20.　Which of the following is **unrelated** to the glossopharyngeal nerve? (　　)

A.　Otic ganglion

B.　Pterygopalatine ganglion

C.　Superior ganglion

D.　Inferior ganglion

21.　Which of the following is related the glossopharyngeal nerve? (　　)

A.　Otic ganglion

B.　Pterygopalatine ganglion

C.　Submandibular ganglion

D.　Geniculate ganglion

22.　Which of the following statements about glossopharyngeal nerve is true? (　　)

A.　It passes through the jugular foramen.

B.　It controls the secretion of the submandibular gland.

C.　It contains the general somatic motor fibers.

D.　It contains the special somatic sensory fibers.

23. Which of the following statements about glossopharyngeal nerve is **not** true? (   )
    A. It passes through the jugular foramen.
    B. It controls the secretion of the parotid gland.
    C. It contains the general somatic motor fibers.
    D. It contains the general somatic sensory fibers.

24. Which of the following conveys the sensation on the carotid sinus? (   )
    A. Facial nerve
    B. Glossopharyngeal nerve
    C. Trigeminal nerve
    D. Vagus nerve

25. The following nerves contain the special visceral motor fibers **except** (   ).
    A. trigeminal nerve
    B. facial nerve
    C. vagus nerve
    D. maxillary nerve

26. Which of the following contains the general visceral motor fibers? (   )
    A. Trigeminal nerve
    B. Oculomotor nerve
    C. Maxillary nerve
    D. Hypoglossal nerve

27. Which of the following statements about the vagus nerve is true? (   )
    A. It contains the general visceral sensory fibers.
    B. It controls the secretion of the sublingual gland.
    C. It passes through the stylohyoid foramen.
    D. It contains the special visceral sensory fibers.

28. Which of the following innervates the cricothyroid? (   )
    A. Internal laryngeal nerve
    B. Inferior laryngeal nerve
    C. Recurrent laryngeal nerve
    D. External laryngeal nerve

29. Which of the following statements about the superior laryngeal nerve is true?
    (   )
    A. It is divided into the internal and external laryngeal nerves.
    B. It conveys the sensory on the mucous membrane of the larynx below the vocal folds.
    C. It innervates all the muscles except the cricothyroid.
    D. It contains special visceral sensory and special visceral motor fibers.

30. Which of the following statements about the recurrent laryngeal nerve is **not** true?
    (   )

A. It contains general visceral sensory and special visceral motor fibers.

B. Its terminal branch is the inferior laryngeal nerve.

C. It innervates all the muscles except the cricothyroid.

D. The right recurrent laryngeal nerve hooks around the aortic arch.

31. Where does the accessory nerve leave the cranium? (   )

A. Foreman lacerum

B. Jugular foramen

C. Foreman magnum

D. Hypoglossal canal

32. Which of the following is **unrelated** to the tongue? (   )

A. Trigeminal nerve

B. Facial nerve

C. Glossopharyngeal nerve

D. Accessory nerve

33. Which of the following is **unrelated** to the sensation of tongue? (   )

A. Trigeminal nerve

B. Facial nerve

C. Hypoglossal nerve

D. Glossopharyngeal nerve

34. Which of the following is **not** supplied by hypoglossal nerves? (   )

A. Intrinsic muscles of tongue

B. Genioglossus

C. Digastric

D. Hyoglossus

35. Which of the following supplies the masticatory muscles? (   )

A. Maxillary nerve

B. Mandibular nerve

C. Facial nerve

D. Zygomatic nerve

36. Which of the following is distributed to the cornea? (   )

A. Optic nerve

B. Nasociliary nerve

C. Lacrimal nerve

D. Frontal nerve

37. Which of the following conveys the sensation of the external acoustic meatus?

(   )

A. Greater auricular nerve

B. Facial nerve

C. Vestibulocochlear nerve

D. Vagus nerve

38. Which of the following conveys the sensation of the parotid gland? (   )

    A. Auriculotemporal nerve

    B. Zygomatic nerve

    C. Glossopharyngeal nerve

    D. Pterygopalatine nerve

39. Which of the following controls the secretion of the parotid gland? (   )

    A. Vagus nerve

    B. Facial nerve

    C. Glossopharyngeal nerve

    D. Buccal nerve

40. Which of the following controls the secretion of the lacrimal gland? (   )

    A. Zygomatic nerve

    B. Facial nerve

    C. Lacrimal nerve

    D. Frontal nerve

II. Double choices(Choose the two best answers among the following choices, and write down the corresponding letters in bracket)

1. Two types of fibers in the trigeminal nerve are (   )

    A. special visceral motor fibers

    B. general visceral sensory fibers

    C. special visceral sensory fibers

    D. general somatic motor fibers

    E. general somatic sensory fibers

2. Which ones of the following are related to the facial nerve? (   )

    A. Ciliary ganglion

    B. Submandibular ganglion

    C. Pterygopalatine ganglion

    D. Otic ganglion

    E. Superior ganglion

3. Which ones of the following convey the taste sensation of the tongue? (   )

    A. Lingual nerve

    B. Hypoglossal nerve

    C. Glossopharyngeal nerve

    D. Facial nerve

    E. Vagus nerve

4. The major terminal branches of the left vagus nerve in the abdomen are (   )

    A. anterior gastric branch

    B. posterior gastric branch

    C. hepatic branch

    D. celiac branch

    E. branch of fundus of stomach

5. Which ones of the following do **not** pass through the jugular foreman? (　　)

    A. Hypoglossal nerve

    B. Facial nerve

    C. Vagus nerve

    D. Accessory nerve

    E. Glossopharyngeal nerve

6. Which ones of the following are **unrelated** to the sensation of tongue? (　　)

    A. Mandibular nerve

    B. Hypoglossal nerve

    C. Glossopharyngeal nerve

    D. Facial nerve

    E. Vagus nerve

7. Which ones of the following are innervated by accessory nerve? (　　)

    A. Platysma

    B. Digastric

    C. Sternocleidomastoid

    D. Trapezius

    E. Omohyoid

8. Which ones of the following do **not** contain the special visceral sensory fibers? (　　)

    A. Trigeminal nerve

    B. Facial nerve

    C. Glossopharyngeal nerve

    D. Optic nerve

    E. Olfactory nerve

9. Which ones of the following are related to the general visceral motor fibers? (　　)

    A. Superior ganglion

    B. Intramural ganglia

    C. Inferior ganglion

    D. Paramural ganglia

    E. Trigeminal ganglion

10. Which ones of the following are related to the sensation of the cerebral dura mater?

    (　　)

    A. Trigeminal nerve

    B. Optic nerve

    C. Vagus nerve

D. Accessory nerve

E. Glossopharyngeal nerve

11. Which ones of the following statements about the hypoglossal nerve are true?
( )

A. It is a special visceral motor nerve.

B. It passes through the jugular foramen.

C. Injury to the hypoglossal nerve results in paralysis of the affected side of the tongue.

D. It innervates the muscles of tongue

E. It innervates the digastric

12. Which ones of the following statements about the olfactory nerve are **not** true?
( )

A. Its fibers are from the neurons in the olfactory bulb.

B. It is composed of the peripheral process given off by the olfactory cells.

C. It is a special visceral sensory nerve.

D. It is distributed on the mucous membrane of the olfactory region.

E. The olfactory filaments pierce the cribriform foramina and enter the cranium.

13. Which ones of the following are innervated by trigeminal nerve? ( )

A. Anterior belly of the digastric

B. Geniohyoid

C. Mylohyoid

D. Genioglossus

E. Superior belly of the omohyoid

14. The fibers in the chorda tympani nerve include ( ).

A. the general visceral sensory fibers

B. the special visceral sensory fibers

C. the general visceral motor fibers

D. the special visceral motor fibers

E. the general somatic sensory fibers

15. Which ones of the following belong to the parasympathetic ganglia? ( )

A. Geniculate ganglion

B. Intramural ganglia

C. Inferior ganglion

D. Cochlear ganglion

E. Otic ganglion

Ⅲ. Fill the blanks (Fill the most appropriate words in the blanks)

1. The optic nerve originates from the _____ cells of the retina and passes through the _____ into the _____ cranial fossa.

2. The nerves passing through the superior orbital fissure are _____ , _____ ,
     _____ and _____ .

3. The nerves passing through the jugular foreman are _____ , _____ , and

     _____ .

4. The parasympathetic fibers in the oculomotor nerve end in _____ ganglion
    which gives off the postganglionic fibers to supply the _____ and _____ .

5. The trigeminal nerve contains _____ and _____ fibers, and its three divi-
    sions are _____ , _____ and _____ .

6. The parasympathetic ganglia related to the facial nerve are _____ and _____
    which give off the postganglionic fibers supplying the _____ , _____ , and
    _____ glands.

7. The branches of facial outside the facial canal are _____ , _____ , _____
    ___ , _____ and _____ .

8. The vestibulocochlear nerve contains _____ fibers, and the ganglia related to it
    are _____ and _____ .

9. The glossopharyngeal nerve passes through _____ leaving the cranium, and the
    ganglia related to it is _____ which give off the postganglionic fibers supplying
    the _____ gland.

10. The vagus nerve contains _____ , _____ , _____ , and _____
     fibers.

11. The anterior vagal trunk is divided into _____ and _____ two major ter-
     minal branches, and the posterior vagal trunk is divided into _____ and ____
     _____ two major terminal branches.

12. The superior obliquus is innervated by _____ nerve, the lateral rectus is inner-
     vated by _____ nerve and the inferior obliquus is innervated by _____
     nerve.

13. The nerves conveying the taste sensation of tongue are the _____ nerve of the
     facial nerve and _____ branch of the glossopharyngeal nerve.

14. The accessory nerve contains _____ fibers, and passes through the _____
     leaving the cranium to supply the _____ and _____ .

15. The hypoglossal nerve contains _____ fibers, and passes through the _____
     ____ leaving the cranium.

IV. Answer questions briefly

1. Please describe the name and innervation nerves of the extraocular muscles.

2. Please briefly describe the name of the two trunks and their terminal branches of va-
    gus nerve in the abdomen, respectively.

3. Please briefly describe the name of cranial nerves that contain the general visceral
    motor fibers and its paraganglia.

4. Please briefly describe the name of cranial nerves that only contain one type of motor fibers.

5. Please briefly describe the name of cranial nerves that control the sensation and motor of tongue.

6. Please briefly describe the name of 5 branches and the corresponding effectors of facial nerve which innervate facial muscles.

7. Please list the special visceral sensory and briefly describe the name of cranial nerves which control special visceral sensory respectively.

8. Please briefly describe the name of cranial nerves that control masticatory muscles and muscles of pharynx and larynx.

Ⅴ. Answer questions in detail

1. Please describe the name, the fibrous components and the classification of the cranial nerves.

2. Please describe the name and corresponding nerve of the parasympathetic ganglia of cranial nerves. And list the muscles or glands controlled by their postganglionic parasympathetic fibers, respectively.

3. Please describe the passages of the 12 pairs of cranial nerves in or out the skull.

Ⅵ. Problems in life

1. Why do you cough when your ear is probed?

2. Do the vestibular organs work during space travel?

Chapter 25　The Visceral Nervous System

Ⅰ. **Single choice（Choose the best answer among the following four choices，and write down the corresponding letter in bracket）**

1. Which of the following statements is true about sympathetic nerve? （　）
   A. The lower center is located in the brainstem and spinal cord.
   B. Sympathetic ganglia has paraorganic and intraorganic ganglia.
   C. The greater splanchnic nerve is composed of postganglionic fibers.
   D. Gray communicating branches are postganglionic fibers and return to the spinal nerves.

2. About the sympathetic trunk, which statement is correct? （　）
   A. It is composed of paravertebral ganglia and interganglionic branches.
   B. The coccygeal ganglion is in front of the coccygeal vertebra.
   C. The cervical sympathetic trunk has only one ganglion.
   D. All ganglia of sympathetic trunk have white communicating branches connected with spinal nerves.

3. Regarding parasympathetic nerve, which is the correct statement? （　）
   A. The lower center is located in the brainstem only.
   B. There are gray and white communicating branches connected to the spinal nerves.
   C. There are paraorganic ganglia and intraorganic ganglia.
   D. Preganglionic fibers are short and postganglionic fibers are long.

4. The preganglionic fibers of greater splanchnic nerve terminate mainly at （　）.
   A. superior mesenteric ganglion
   B. inferior mesenteric ganglion
   C. celiac ganglion
   D. aorticorenal ganglion

5. Which of the following does **not** belong to the parasympathetic ganglia in skull?
   （　）
   A. Ciliary ganglion
   B. Trigeminal ganglion
   C. Otic ganglion
   D. Submandibular ganglion

6. The parasympathetic postganglionic fibers innervating the parotid gland originate from （　）.
   A. inferior salivary nucleus
   B. geniculate ganglion

    C. otic ganglion

    D. pterygopalatine ganglion

7. Cranial nerves containing parasympathetic preganglionic fibers are (   ).

    A. Ⅲ、Ⅶ、Ⅸ、Ⅹ

    B. Ⅲ、Ⅶ、Ⅸ、Ⅺ

    C. Ⅴ、Ⅶ、Ⅸ、Ⅹ

    D. Ⅲ、Ⅷ、Ⅸ、Ⅹ

8. Which one belongs to paravertebral ganglia of the sympathetic nerve? (   )

    A. Superior mesenteric ganglion

    B. Inferior mesenteric ganglion

    C. Celiac ganglion

    D. Impar ganglion

9. The lower center of sympathetic nerve is located in (   ).

    A. $T_1 - L_3$ segments of spinal cord

    B. $T_1 - T_{12}$ segments of spinal cord

    C. $S_2 - S_4$ segments of spinal cord

    D. $T_1 - S_3$ segments of spinal cord

10. About the communicating branch of sympathetic nerve, which one is **false**? (   )

    A. There are white and gray communicating branches.

    B. The white communicating branch consists of preganglionic fibers.

    C. The gray communicating branch consists of postganglionic fibers.

    D. All thoracic and lumbar nerves connect to the sympathetic trunk by white communicating branches.

11. The greater and lesser splanchnic nerves contain (   ).

    A. sympathetic postganglionic fibers

    B. sympathetic preganglionic fibers

    C. parasympathetic postganglionic fibers

    D. parasympathetic preganglionic fibers

12. Which one contains sympathetic postganglionic fibers as follow? (   )

    A. Greater splanchnic nerve

    B. lesser splanchnic nerve

    C. Lumbar splanchnic nerve

    D. Femoral nerve

13. Which one contains parasympathetic preganglionic fibers as follow? (   )

    A. Greater splanchnic nerve

    B. Lesser splanchnic nerve,

    C. Lumbar splanchnic nerve

    D. Pelvic splanchnic nerve

14. Which one belongs to parasympathetic ganglia? (   )

A. Ganglion in cardiac plexus

B. Trigeminal ganglion

C. Celiac ganglion

D. Superior mesenteric ganglion

15. Which one belongs to sympathetic ganglia? (   )

A. Ciliary ganglion

B. Pterygopalatine ganglion

C. Submandibular ganglion

D. Celiac ganglion

16. The ganglion associated with secretion of the lacrimal gland is (   ).

A. ciliary ganglion

B. otic ganglion

C. pterygopalatine ganglion

D. submandibular ganglion

17. Postganglionic fibers that control the secretion of the sublingual gland come from

(   ).

A. ciliary ganglion

B. otic ganglion

C. pterygopalatine ganglion

D. submandibular ganglion

18. Parasympathetic nuclei in the brain stem do **not** include (   ).

A. accessory nucleus of oculomotor nerve

B. nucleus ambiguous

C. inferior salivary nucleus

D. superior salivary nucleus

19. Which one does **not** belong to sympathetic nerve? (   )

A. Greater splanchnic nerve

B. Lesser splanchnic nerve

C. Lumbar splanchnic nerve

D. Pelvic splanchnic nerve

20. Parasympathetic fibers of the oculomotor nerve innervate (   ).

A. dilator pupillae

B. parotid gland

C. sphincter pupillae

D. sublingual gland

Ⅱ. **Double choices (Choose the two best answers among the following choices, and write down the corresponding letters in bracket)**

1. Which ones of the following are the correct descriptions of sympathetic nerve?

(   )

A. The lower center is in the spinal cord of $C_8 - L_2$.

B. The number of paravertebral ganglia is the same as that of vertebrae.

C. The white communicating branches are preganglionic fibers, only seen in 15 pairs of spinal nerves.

D. All preganglionic fibers enter the paravertebral ganglia.

E. All preganglionic fibers make rely at the paravertebral ganglia.

2. The lower center of sympathetic nerve is located in (   ).

A. thoracic and lumbar segments of spinal cord

B. S_{2-4} segments of spinal cord

C. lateral horn of gray matter of the spinal cord

D. $T_1 - L_3$ segments of spinal cord

E. brainstem and sacral spinal cord

3. Descriptions of sympathetic trunk, which ones of the following are correct? (   )

A. It lies on both sides of the vertebral column.

B. It is composed of paravertebral ganglia and interganglionic branches.

C. White communicating branches are preganglionic fibers, 31 pairs.

D. Gray communicating branches are preganglionic fibers, 31 pairs.

E. It does not connect to the spinal nerves.

4. Sympathetic ganglia include (   ).

A. ciliary ganglion

B. celiac ganglion

C. pterygopalatine ganglion

D. middle cervical ganglion

E. otic ganglion

5. Descriptions of parasympathetic nerve, which ones of the following are correct? (   ).

A. S_{2-4} segments of spinal cord have parasympathetic center.

B. Celiac ganglion belongs to parasympathetic ganglion.

C. It controls the sphincter pupillae and ciliary muscle.

D. Preganglionic fibers are short and postganglionic fibers are long.

E. It belongs to visceral afferent nerves.

6. The lower center of parasympathetic nerve is located in (   ).

A. lateral part of the intermediate zone of the $T_1 - L_3$ segments of the spinal cord

B. lateral part of the intermediate zone of the S_{2-4} segments of the spinal cord

C. oculomotor nucleus, facial nucleus, superior salivary nucleus and inferior salivary nucleus

D. E-W nucleus, superior salivary nucleus, inferior salivary nucleus and dorsal nucleus of vagus nerve

E. red nucleus and substantia nigra

7. Which ones of the following belong to parasympathetic ganglia? (   )

A. Trigeminal ganglion

B. Geniculate ganglion

C. Pterygopalatine ganglion

D. Submandibular ganglion

E. Superior cervical ganglion

8. The characteristics of parasympathetic nerve, which ones of the following are correct? (   )

A. Preganglionic fiber are long.

B. Preganglionic fibers are short.

C. Its distribution is wide.

D. Its distribution is limited.

E. It does not form the visceral nervous plexus.

Ⅲ. Fill the blanks (Fill the most appropriate words in the blanks)

1. The visceral motor nerves include _____ and _____.

2. The lower center of sympathetic nerve is located in _____.

3. There are two types of sympathetic ganglia, named _____ and _____.

4. Sympathetic trunk consists of _____ and _____.

5. The lower center of the parasympathetic nerve is located in _____ and _____.

6. Parasympathetic ganglia in the skull include _____, _____, _____ and _____.

7. Parasympathetic nuclei in the brainstem include _____, _____, _____ and _____.

8. The communicating branches of sympathetic nerve are _____ and _____.

Ⅳ. Answer questions briefly

1. Please describe the position of the lower center of sympathetic nerve and the sympathetic ganglia.

2. Please describe the position of lower center of parasympathetic nerve and parasympathetic ganglia

3. Please describe the concept and direction of sympathetic preganglionic fibers.

4. What are the parasympathetic nuclei in the brainstem?

5. What is the greater splanchnic nerve and the lesser splanchnic nerve?

Ⅴ. Answer questions in detail

1. Please describe the lower center and ganglia of the sympathetic and parasympathetic nerves.

2. Please describe the origin and relay of the parasympathetic preganglionic fibers in the lacrimal gland and the salivary glands.

VI. Problems in life

When you see your favorite food, why are your digestive juices begin to flow?

Part 6 The Endocrine Organs

Ⅰ. **Single choice（Choose the best answer among the following four choices, and write down the corresponding letter in bracket）**

1. Which of the characteristics of endocrine glands is **wrong**? （　　）
    A. It has not output duct.
    B. Blood supply is rich.
    C. It is small size and light weight.
    D. Secretions are discharged into the lumen of the human body and can be collected.

2. Which of the following endocrine organ is located in cranial cavity? （　　）
    A. Pituitary gland
    B. Thyroid gland
    C. Hypothalamus
    D. Epithalamus

3. Which of the following organs is both an endocrine and a lymphatic organ? （　　）
    A. Pituitary gland
    B. Thyroid gland
    C. Thymus
    D. Spleen

4. In addition to the gonads, the organ that secretes sex hormones is （　　）.
    A. islets of pancreas
    B. suprarenal gland
    C. thymus
    D. pineal body

5. Which of the following organs does **not** belong to endocrine glands? （　　）
    A. Pituitary gland
    B. Thyroid
    C. Prostate
    D. Thymus

6. Which of the following organs can cause the decrease of serum calcium due to insufficient secretion? （　　）
    A. Pineal body
    B. Thyroid gland
    C. Parathyroid gland
    D. Gonad

7. Which of the following glands enlargement can cause by iodine deficiency? (   )

   A. Hypophysis

   B. Thyroid gland

   C. Parathyroid gland

   D. Thymus

8. Which of the following description of the adrenal gland is **wrong**? (   )

   A. It is located in the retroperitoneal space.

   B. It is an extraperitoneal organ.

   C. The left one is semilunar shape.

   D. The right one is semilunar shape.

9. Which is **wrong** about the descriptions of pituitary gland? (   )

   A. It is located in the anterior cranial fossa.

   B. It is connected to the hypothalamus through the infundibulum.

   C. Anterior lobes called adenohypophysis and can secretes many hormones.

   D. Posterior lobe called the neurohypophysis, which stores hormones only.

10. Which of the following structures can secret thyrotropin? (   )

    A. Anterior lobe of pituitary gland

    B. Posterior lobe of pituitary gland

    C. Thyroid gland

    D. Parathyroid gland

11. About the adenohypophysis, which one is correct? (   )

    A. It includes the distal, nodule and intermediate parts.

    B. It is composed of infundibulum and nervous part.

    C. It can be called anterior lobe.

    D. It can secret the oxytocin.

12. About the neurohypophysis, which one is correct? (   )

    A. It consists of the distal, nodule and intermediate parts.

    B. It secrets somatotropin.

    C. It includes anterior and posterior lobes.

    D. It includes nervous part and infundibulum.

13. Which one is the correct description of the pineal gland? (   )

    A. Excessive secretion promotes sexual precocity.

    B. Excessive secretion can cause delayed puberty.

    C. It is underdeveloped in childhood.

    D. It secrets sex hormones.

14. Which one is the correct description of thymus? (   )

    A. It secrets thymosin.

    B. It secrets thymopoietin.

    C. It is developed in old age.

  D. It belongs to immune organs.
15. Diabetes results from the shortage of (   ).
  A. glucagon
  B. insulin
  C. glucocorticoid
  D. melatonin

II. Double choices(Choose the two best answers among the following choices, and write down the corresponding letters in bracket)

  1. Which ones of the characteristics that do **not** belong to endocrine glands? (   )
    A. It has not output duct.
    B. Blood supply is poor.
    C. It is small size and lightweight.
    D. Secretions are powerful.
    E. It is not dominated by the nervous system.
  2. Which ones of the descriptions of thyroid gland are correct? (   )
    A. It is divided into isthmus and pyramidal lobe only.
    B. The isthmus lies in front of the cricoid cartilage.
    C. The isthmus lies in front of the 2−4 tracheal cartilage ring.
    D. The pyramidal lobe lies on both sides.
    E. The parathyroid gland is behind lateral lobe.
  3. The organs secreting sex hormones are (   ).
    A. pituitary gland
    B. pineal body
    C. thyroid gland
    D. gonad gland
    E. adrenal gland
  4. Which ones of the following statements about hormones are **wrong**? (   )
    A. It is secreted by ductal glands.
    B. It enters to blood flow directly.
    C. It is secreted by ductless gland.
    D. It is less quantity and greater effect.
    E. It is not related to the nervous system.
  5. About the suprarenal gland, which ones are correct? (   )
    A. It is located in the retroperitoneal space.
    B. It is an intraperitoneal organ.
    C. Left adrenal gland is triangular shape.
    D. Right adrenal gland is semilunar shape.
    E. The hormones secreted contain sex hormones.

III. Fill the blanks (Fill the most appropriate words in the blanks)

1. The endocrine system consists of _____ and _____.
2. The substance secreted by endocrine organ is called _____.
3. The endocrine organs in the cranial cavity are _____ and _____.
4. According to the structures, the hypophysis is subdivided into two parts: _____ and _____.
5. The hormones stored in neurohypophysis are secreted by _____.
6. In the neck, endocrine organs are _____ and _____.
7. The thyroid gland is butterfly-shaped consisting of _____ and _____, in addition, it has _____ in some body.
8. The endocrine organ in the chest is _____.
9. About the shape of suprarenal gland, the left one is _____, the right one is _____.
10. The insulin is secreted by _____ in pancreas.

IV. Answer questions briefly

1. What is endocrine gland? Which organs are included?
2. Please describe the location, division and general function of pituitary gland.
3. Please describe the position and features of thyroid gland.
4. Please describe the location, shape and artery of suprarenal gland.

V. Answer questions in detail

Please describe the characteristics of endocrine system.

VI. Problems in life

1. Does milk production cease once the menstrual cycle resumes after pregnancy?
2. What is goiter?

Answers

Part 1   The Locomotor System

Chapter 1   The Bones

I. **Single choice**

1. D	2. C	3. B	4. A	5. B	6. B	7. C	8. D	9. D	10. D
11. D	12. B	13. A	14. C	15. B	16. C	17. C	18. C	19. A	20. B
21. B	22. A	23. C	24. D	25. B	26. B	27. D	28. C	29. A	30. D
31. C	32. D	33. A	34. C	35. B	36. D	37. C	38. C	39. B	40. D
41. B	42. B	43. B	44. D	45. C	46. A	47. A	48. C	49. D	50. B
51. D	52. B	53. D	54. D	55. D	56. D				

II. **Double choices**

1. AD	2. BE	3. CE	4. CE	5. CE	6. CE	7. BD	8. AE	9. AB
10. BD	11. BC	12. BD	13. AE	14. BC	15. BC	16. CE	17. AE	18. DE
19. CE	20. BE							

III. **Fill the blanks**

1. skull, bones of trunk
2. long bone, short bone, flat bone, irregular bone
3. compact bone, spongy bone
4. fibrous membrane, vascular membrane
5. red marrow, yellow marrow
6. vertebra, sternum, rib
7. eighth, ninth, tenth
8. manubrium, body, xiphoid process
9. scapula, clavicle
10. carpal bones, metacarpal bones, phalanges
11. ilium, pubis, ischium
12. intertrochanteric line, intertrochanteric crest
13. vertebral body, vertebral arch, vertebral foramen
14. frontal bone, occipital bone, ethmoid bone, sphenoid bone
15. zygomatic process of temporal bone, temporal process of zygomatic bone

16. foramen rotundum, foramen ovale, foramen spinosum

17. coronoid process, condylar process

18. body, greater wings, lesser wings, pterygoid processes

19. horizontal plate, perpendicular plate, horizontal plate

20. frontal process, zygomatic process, alveolar process, palatine process

IV. Answer questions briefly

1. According to the shape, bones are classified into the long, short, flat and irregular bones. Long bone consists of a shaft and two extremities. They distribute in limbs. Short bones are roughly in cuboid shape. They distribute in wrist and foot such as the carpal and tarsal bones. Flat bones consist of two plates of compact bone with spongy bone between them. They include the ribs, sternum, scapula, and many bones of the skull. Irregular bones vary greatly in shape. They include many of the cranial bones, vertebrae, and the hip bone. Some cranial bones containing air-filled cavities are pneumatic bones.

2. Living bones consist of bony substance, periosteum, bone marrow, blood and nerve supply. Bony substance includes compact bone and spongy bone. Periosteum consists of two layers: an outer or fibrous layer and an inner or vascular membrane. Bone marrow consists of two types, red marrow and yellow marrow.

3. A typical vertebra is made up of two principal parts, the anterior vertebral body and posterior vertebral arch. They enclose vertebral foramen. All of the vertebral foramina form the vertebral canal. The vertebral arch has a pair of pedicles and a pair of laminae. There are seven processes extending from the vertebral arch, including a pair of transverse processes, a pair of superior articular processes, a pair of inferior articular processes, and a spinous process. Above and below the vertebral pedicle, there are the superior and inferior vertebral notches. The adjacent superior and inferior vertebral notches enclose an intervertebral foramen.

4. The main characteristics of cervical vertebrae are: transverse foramen in each transverse process; small vertebral body; the vertebral foramen is relatively large nearly triangular in shape; the spines are short and bifid except the first and seventh; the articular facets are relatively horizontal.

5. The thoracic vertebrae are mainly characterized by two costal facets on each side of their bodies. The spines are long and slop downwards, the articular facets of articular processes are relatively coronal. The vertebral body is heart-shaped and the vertebral foramen is nearly circular and smaller than that in other regions.

6. Lumbar vertebrae are large. The vertebral body is kidney-shaped and the vertebral foramen is triangular. The spines are thick, quadrilateral and horizontal. The articular facets of articular processes are relatively sagittal.

7. The scapula is a triangular flat bone. It has three borders (the medial, lateral and superior borders), three angles (the superior, inferior and lateral angles), and two

surfaces (the anterior and posterior surfaces). The medial border is vertebral border and the lateral border is axillary border. The superior border has scapular notch and coracoid process. The superior and inferior angles are opposite to the second and seventh ribs relatively. The lateral angle is thick and has an articular surface, the glenoid cavity. The anterior surface is subscapular fossa. The posterior surface is divided into supraspinous and infraspinous fossae by the spine of scapula.

8. The mandible consists of one body and two rami. The body has two borders (superior and inferior borders) and two surfaces (the internal and external surfaces). The upper border is alveolar arch, and lower border is the base of mandible. The ramus of mandible is a square plate of bone. There are two processes on its superior end, the anterior one is corocoid process, posterior one is the condylar process with the head of mandible. The constricted portion below the head is the neck of mandible. Between the two processes is the mandibular notch. The portion where the body meet the ramus is mandibular angle.

9. It is the longest and heaviest bone in the body and consists of a shaft and two ends. The upper end comprises a head, a neck and two trochanters (the greater and lesser trochanters). Near the center of head, there is the fovea of femoral head. Between the two trochanters, there are intertrochanteric line on the anterior surface and the intertrochanteric crest on the posterior surface. The shaft of femur is convex slightly forward. There are linea aspera, gluteal tuberosity, and pectineal line on the back of shaft. The lower end is expanded and includes the medial and lateral condyles, medial and lateral epicondyles, patellar surface, intercondylar fossa and adductor tubercle.

10. The skull may be divided into two types of bones: cerebral cranium and facial cranium. The cerebral cranium consists of eight cranial bones. They are one frontal bone, one occipital bone, one ethmoid bone, one sphenoid bone, two parietal bones and two temporal bones. The facial cranium consists of fifteen facial bones. They are two palatine bones, two zygomatic bones, two nasal bones, two lacrimal bones, two inferior nasal conchae, two maxillae, one vomer, one mandible, and one hyoid bone.

V. Answer questions in detail

1. Shape and structures: The orbit is shaped roughly like a four-sided pyramid. It has an apex, a base and four walls. The optic canal is situated at the apex, opens posteromedially to the middle cranial fossa. The superior wall is formed by the orbital plate of the frontal bone and the lesser wings of sphenoid bone. Anterolaterally, there is the lacrimal fossa for the lacrimal gland. At the middle part of the supraorbital margin presents the supraorbital notch or supraorbital foramen. The lateral wall is thickest. The superior and inferior orbital fissures separate the lateral wall from the superior and inferior walls relatively. The inferior wall is thin and forms the roof of maxillary sinus. The infraorbital groove runs forward, passes through the infraorbital canal,

and ends in the infraorbital foramen, which lies 0.5 – 1.0 cm below the infraorbital margin. The medial wall is the thinnest and formed mainly by the orbital plate of the ethmoid bone. Anteroinferiorly, there is the fossa for lacrimal sac.

Communications: Through the optic canal and superior orbital fissure, the orbit communicates with the middle cranial fossa. Through the inferior orbital fissure, the orbit communicates with the infratemporal fossa and pterygopalatine fossa. Through the infraorbital groove and infraorbital canal, the orbit opens to the infraorbital foramen. Through the fossa for lacrimal sac and nasolacrimal canal, the orbit opens to the nasal cavity.

2. Formation: The middle cranial fossa consists of a narrow median portion formed by the body of the sphenoid bone and two deeply concave lateral portions formed by the greater wings of the sphenoid bone with the squamous and petrous parts of the temporal bone.

Main structures: On the upper surface of the body of sphenoid bone, there are the anterior clinoid processes, sulcus prechiasmaticus, hypophysial fossa, carotid sulcus and dorsum sellae of sphenoid bone. Posterior to the carotid sulcus is the foramen lacerum. Superior orbital fissure lies between the lesser and greater wings of sphenoid bone. On the root of greater wings of sphenoid bone, there are three pairs of foramina, the foramen rotundum, foramen ovale and foramen spinosum. At the apex and anterior aspect of the petrous part of temporal bone, there are the trigeminal impression, arcuate eminence, and tegmen tympani.

Communications: The optic canal and superior orbital fissure communicate with the orbit. The foramen rotundum opens into the pterygopalatine fossa. The foramen ovale and foramen spinosum open into the infratemporal fossa.

3. The paranasal sinuses distribute around the nasal cavity, and include the frontal sinus, ethmoidal sinus, sphenoidal sinus and the maxillary sinus.

Frontal sinus: The two frontal sinuses are contained in the frontal bone deeper to the glabella and superciliary arch, and separated by a septum. Each sinus opens into the anterior part of the middle nasal meatus of the nasal cavity.

Ethmoidal sinus: They lie in the ethmoidal labyrinth, and can be divided into three groups. The anterior and middle groups open into the middle nasal meatus of the nasal cavity; the posterior group opens into the superior nasal meatus of the nasal cavity.

Sphenoidal sinus: They are contained in the body of the sphenoid bone and separated by a thin bony plate. Each sinus opens into the sphenoethmoidal recess.

Maxillary sinus: They are the largest paranasal sinuses locating in the body of maxillae. Each sinus communicates with the middle nasal meatus of the nasal cavity.

4. Bony nasal cavities are irregular spaces which extend from the roof of the mouth to the base of the cranial cavity, and are separated from each other by a bony nasal sep-

tum. There are a single anterior nasal aperture (piriform aperture) and a pair of posterior nasal apertures.

Each bony nasal cavity contains a roof, a floor, a lateral wall and a medial wall. The roof is mainly formed by the cribriform plate of the ethmoid bone. The floor is the hard palate formed by the maxilla and the palatine bone. The lateral wall is formed by the maxilla, lacrimal bone, inferior nasal concha, ethmoidal labyrinth, perpendicular plate of the palatine bone and the pterygoid process of sphenoid bone. On the lateral wall, there are superior, middle and inferior nasal conchae and superior, middle and inferior nasal meatuses. The medial wall is the bony nasal septum that is formed by the vomer and the perpendicular plate of the ethmoid bone.

5. The hip bone is formed by the fusion of three components: the ilium, pubis and ischium. The area of fusion is the acetabulum. There are acetabular notch, lunate surface and acetabular fossa in the acetabulum.

The ilium consists of a body and an ala. The body forms the upper two-fifths of the acetabulum. The superior border of the ala is iliac crest. It ends anterior superior iliac spine and posterior superior iliac spine. Below these two spines are the anterior inferior iliac spine and posterior inferior iliac spine respectively. Inferior to the posterior inferior iliac spine is the greater sciatic notch. The prominent projection on the outer lip of the iliac crest is the tubercle of iliac crest. The internal surface of the iliac ala is iliac fossa. Its inferior border is arcuate line. Posteroinferior to the iliac fossa, there is the auricular surface that articulates with the sacrum.

The ischium comprises a body and a ramus. The body forms the posterior two-fifths of the acetabulum. In the lower end of the body, there is the ischial tuberosity. Ischial spine is the triangle projection extending from the posterior border of the body. It separates the greater sciatic notch superiorly from the lesser sciatic notch inferiorly. The ramus projects forward and upward from the ischial tuberosity to join the inferior ramus of pubis.

The pubis comprises a body and two rami, superior ramus and inferior ramus. The body fuses with the ischium and ilium and forms the anteroinferior one-fifth part of the acetabulum. On the upper border of the superior ramus, there are pectin pubis, pubic tubercle, and pubic crest. The inferior ramus passes backward, downward to join the ramus of ischium. The bodies and rami of pubis and ischium form an oval space, the obturator foramen. Between the two rami, there is the pubic symphysis.

Chapter 2   The Joints

I . **Single choice**

1. D	2. B	3. A	4. D	5. B	6. B	7. A	8. B	9. C	10. B
11. A	12. D	13. B	14. D	15. B	16. A	17. B	18. C	19. A	20. C
21. B	22. D	23. B	24. D	25. A	26. C	27. C	28. B	29. D	30. D

31. D	32. C	33. D	34. D	35. B	36. A	37. C	38. C	39. D	40. C
41. A	42. B	43. D	44. C	45. D	46. D	47. C	48. D	49. B	50. A
51. B	52. D	53. A	54. C	55. D	56. D	57. D	58. D	59. D	60. D

II. Double choices

1. AC	2. BD	3. CE	4. AC	5. BE	6. AC	7. AC	8. BC	9. AE
10. BE	11. CE	12. DE	13. BD	14. CE	15. AE	16. AB	17. AD	18. BC

19. AD   20. AD

III. Fill the blanks

1. fibrous joint, cartilaginous joint, synostosis
2. suture, gomphosis, syndesmosis
3. synchondrosis, symphysis
4. articular surface, articular capsule, articular cavity
5. ligament, articular disc, articular labrum, synovial fold and bursa
6. hinge joint, pivot joint
7. ellipsoid joint, saddle joint
8. ball and socket joint, plane joint
9. tubercle of the rib, transverse process
10. 12 thoracic vertebrae, 12 pairs of ribs with their costal cartilages, sternum
11. annulus fibrosus, nucleus pulposus
12. head of the humerus, glenoid cavity of the scapula
13. cervical curvature, thoracic curvature, lumbar curvature, pelvic curvature
14. humeroulnar joint, humeroradial joint, proximal radioulnar joint
15. apex of coccyx, ischial tuberosity, sacrotuberous ligament, pubic arch, lower border of the pubic symphysis
16. lesser sciatic notch, sacrotuberous ligament, sacrospinous ligament
17. head of femur, fossa of acetabulum
18. anterior cruciate ligament, posterior cruciate ligament
19. shoulder joint, hip joint
20. hip joint, knee joint

IV. Answer questions briefly

1. The connection between bones is called the joint. According to the characteristic features, joint can be classified into two types, the synarthrosis and diarthrosis. The synarthrosis occurs between bones that come into close contact with one another, which include the fibrous joint, cartilaginous joint and synostosis. The diarthrosis is the freely movable articulation. It is called the synovial joint. It has articular surfaces, articular capsule and articular cavity.

2. The essential structures of a synovial joint contain articular surface, articular capsule and articular cavity. The articular surface is covered by the articular cartilage. It contains a convex articular head and a concave articular fossa. The articular capsule is at-

tached to the periphery of the articular surface and the adjacent bone surface. It is composed of an outer layer of fibrous membrane and an inner lining of synovial membrane. The fibrous membrane is dense and rich in blood vessels and nerves. The synovial membrane is thin. It secrets synovial fluid to lubricate the joint. The articular cavity is a closed cavity formed by the synovial membrane and the articular cartilage. It contains a proper amount of synovia, and its pressure is negative to the atmospheric pressure.

3. The accessory structures of a synovial joint contain ligament, articular disc, articular labrum, synovial fold and bursa. Ligament can strengthen and limit the movements of the joint. It can be distributed inside or outside the joint (the intracapsular and extracapsular ligaments). Articular disc is a flattened fibrocartilage between the articular surfaces of the bones. In knee joint, it is semilunar cartilage, the menisci. Articular labrum is a pliable, fibrocartilaginous ring that helps to deepen the articular fossa for the bones. Synovial membrane extends inside or outer the articular cavity to form the synovial fold and synovial bursa.

4. The joints of vertebral bodies contain intervertebral disc, anterior and posterior longitudinal ligaments. The intervertebral disc is a symphysis between vertebral bodies. It consists of a tough, peripheral fibrocartilaginous ring called the annulus fibrosus and a more pliable, inner, gelatinous mass, the nucleus pulposus. The anterior and posterior longitudinal ligaments are long ligaments located in front and behind of the vertebral bodies respectively. They can limit excessive extension and flexion of the vertebral column.

5. The vertebral arches are connected by synovial joints and ligaments. The synovial joint is the zygapophysial joint which lies between the articular processes. The ligaments contain three short ligaments and one long ligament. The short ligaments are ligament flava, interspinal ligament and intertransverse ligament which locate between the adjacent vertebral laminae, spinous processes, and transverse processes respectively. The long ligament is the supraspinal ligament which runs over the tips of the spinous processes and blend with the interspinal ligaments anteriorly.

6. The shoulder joint is a typical ball and socket joint, linking the head of humerus to the glenoid cavity of the scapula. It may do abduction and adduction, flexion and extension, lateral and medial rotation, and circumduction.

7. The elbow joint is a compound synovial joint which contains humeroulnar joint, humeroradial joint and proximal radioulnar joint. The humeroulnar joint is a hinge joint between the trochlea of the humerus and the trochlear notch of the ulna. The humeroradial joint is a ball and socket joint between the capitulum of humerus and the upper concave surface of the radial head. The proximal radioulnar joint is a pivot joint between the head of radius and the radial notch of the ulna. As a whole, the elbow joint is a hinge joint, permitting flexion and extension of the forearm mainly.

8. The hip joint is a typical ball and socket joint, linking the head of femur to the fossa of acetabulum. It permits abduction and adduction, flexion and extension, lateral and medial rotation, and circumduction.

9. The knee joint is the largest and the most complicated joint in the body. It is made up of the joints between the femoral and tibial condyles and between the patella and the patellar surface of the femur. The principal movements of the knee are flexion and extension, but the rotation is possible when the joint is in the flexed position.

10. There are three aspects of the vertebral column as a whole, the anterior, dorsal and lateral aspects. On the anterior aspect, the breadth of vertebral bodies increases from the 2nd cervical to the 2nd sacral, then diminishes rapidly. On the dorsal aspect, the spinous processes project in the midline. The cervical spinous processes are short and bifid. The thoracic spinous processes are long and sloping downward. The lumbar spinous processes are thick and horizontal. On the lateral aspect, there are four physiological curvatures. The thoracic and pelvic curvatures are concave ventrally, and the cervical and lumbar curvatures are convex forwards.

V. Answer questions in detail

1. The essential structures of a synovial joint contain articular surface, articular capsule and articular cavity. The articular surface is covered by the articular cartilage. It contains a convex articular head and a concave articular fossa. The articular capsule is attached to the periphery of the articular surface and the adjacent bone surface. It is composed of an outer layer of fibrous membrane and inner lining of synovial membrane. The fibrous membrane is dense and rich in blood vessels and nerves. The synovial membrane is thin. It secrets synovial fluid to lubricate the joint. The articular cavity is a closed cavity formed by the synovial membrane and the articular cartilage. It contains a proper amount of synovia, and its pressure is negative to the atmospheric pressure.

   The accessory structures of a synovial joint contains ligament, articular disc, articular labrum, synovial fold and bursa. Ligament can strengthen and limit the movements of the joint. It can be distributed inside or outside the joint (the intracapsular and extracapsular ligaments). Articular disc is a flattened fibrocartilage between the articular surfaces of the bones. In knee joint, it is semilunar cartilage, the menisci. Articular labrum is a pliable, fibrocartilaginous ring that helps to deepen the articular surface for the bones. Synovial membrane extends inside or outer the articular cavity to form the synovial fold and synovial bursa. Synovial bursa is a closed, fluid-filled sac. It is continuous with the articular cavity.

2. The articulations of the lumbar vertebrae contain two parts, the joints of vertebral bodies and the joints of vertebral arches.

   The joints of vertebral bodies contain intervertebral disc, anterior and posterior longitudinal ligaments. The intervertebral disc is a symphysis between vertebral bodies. It consists of a tough, peripheral fibrocartilaginous ring called the annulus fibrosus and a more pliable, inner, gelatinous mass, the nucleus pulposus. The anterior and posterior longitudinal ligaments are long ligaments which are located in front and behind of the vertebral bodies respectively. They can limit excessive extension and flexion of the vertebral column.

The joints of vertebral arches contain synovial joints and ligaments. The synovial joint is the zygapophysial joint which lies between the articular processes. The ligaments contain three short ligaments and one long ligament. The short ligaments are ligament flava, interspinal ligament and intertransverse ligament which locate between the adjacent vertebral laminae, spinous processes, and transverse processes respectively. The long ligament is the supraspinal ligament which runs over the tips of the spinous processes and blend with the interspinal ligaments anteriorly.

3. Composition: Shoulder joint is formed by the head of humerus and the glenoid cavity of the scapula.

Characteristics: ①It is a typical ball and socket joint. The articular head is approximately four times larger than the articular fossa. ②There is a glenoid labrum in the articular cavity to deepen the articular fossa. ③The articular capsule is thin and loose, especially in the anteroinferior part. Therefore, the dislocation of the humeral head usually occurs in anteroinferior direction. ④The tendon of the long head of biceps brachii passes through the articular cavity.

Movements: Shoulder joint is a typical ball and socket joint. It may perform abduction and adduction, flexion and extension, lateral and medial rotation, and circumduction.

4. Composition: Hip joint is formed by the head of femur and the fossa of acetabulum.

Characteristics: ①It is a typical ball and socket joint. The head of femur constitutes more than a hemisphere, and about 2/3 is enclosed within the acetabulum. ②There is a acetabular labrum in the articular cavity to deepen the articular fossa. ③The articular capsule is thick and reinforced by ligaments and related muscles. Therefore, the hip joint is more stable and the dislocation of the joint is not common. ④Except for the trochanteric fossa, most of the neck of femur is enclosed in the articular capsule. So, the fracture of femoral neck may be the intracapsular, extracapsular or the mixed type. ⑤The ligament of head of femur connects the acetabular notch and transverse ligament with the fovea of femoral head.

Movements: The hip joint is a typical ball and socket joint. It permits abduction and adduction, flexion and extension, lateral and medial rotation, and circumduction.

5. Composition: Knee joint is made up of the joints between the femoral and tibial condyles and between the patella and the patellar surface of the femur.

Characteristics: ①It is the largest and most complicated joint in the body. ②The articular capsule is reinforced by patellar ligament, oblique popliteal ligament, tibial and fibular collateral ligaments from anterior, posterior, medial and lateral aspects. ③There are two menisci in the articular cavity to deepen the articular surfaces of tibia for the reception of the femoral condyles. ④There are anterior and posterior cruciate ligaments in the articular cavity to stabilize the knee joint. ⑤There are synovial fold and synovial bursa in the articular cavity.

Movements: The principal movements of the knee are flexion and extension, but the rotation is possible when the joint is in the flexed position.

Chapter 3   The Muscles

Ⅰ. **Single choice**

1. C	2. D	3. A	4. D	5. A	6. D	7. A	8. D	9. B	10. C
11. C	12. A	13. D	14. C	15. D	16. C	17. C	18. D	19. A	20. D
21. C	22. D	23. C	24. B	25. C	26. A	27. A	28. A	29. C	30. D
31. A	32. A	33. C	34. B	35. B	36. A	37. A	38. B	39. A	40. A
41. D	42. C	43. D	44. B	45. C	46. C	47. D	48. B	49. B	50. D
51. C	52. C	53. A	54. B	55. B	56. D	57. B	58. C	59. C	60. D

Ⅱ. **Double choices**

1. AD	2. BE	3. AC	4. CD	5. CE	6. AD	7. AE	8. DE	9. AD
10. BC	11. BC	12. AB	13. CE	14. BE	15. CE	16. DE	17. BC	18. DE
19. CE	20. BD							

Ⅲ. **Fill the blanks**

1. long muscle, short muscle, broad muscle, orbicular muscle
2. fascia, synovial bursa, synovial sheath of tendon, sesamoid bone
3. temporalis, masseter, medial pterygoid, lateral pterygoid
4. platysma, sternocleidomastoid
5. Sartorius, quadriceps femoris
6. aortic aperture, esophageal aperture, vena cava aperture
7. digastric, mylohyoid, stylohyoid, geniohyoid
8. sternohyoid, omohyoid, sternothyroid, thyrohyoid
9. obliquus externus abdominis, obliquus internus abdominis, transversus abdominis
10. pectoralis major, pectoralis minor, serratus anterior
11. gastrocnemius, soleus
12. supraglenoid tubercle of scapula, coracoid process of scapula
13. supraspinatus, infraspinatus, teres minor, subscapularis
14. biceps brachii, coracobrachialis, brachialis
15. flexor digitorum superficialis, flexor digitorum profundus
16. psoas major, iliacus
17. rectus femoris, vastus medialis, vastus lateralis, vastus intermedius
18. pectineus, adductor longus, adductor brevis, adductor magnus, gracilis

19. sartorius

20. abdominal aorta, thoracic duct

Ⅳ. **Answer questions briefly**

1. There are three openings in the diaphragm: ① The aortic aperture (hiatus) lies in front of the12th thoracic vertebra. It transmits the abdominal aorta and thoracic duct. ② The esophageal aperture (hiatus) is located in the right crus of the diaphragm at the level of T_{10}. It transmits the esophagus and the anterior and posterior vagal trunks. ③The vena cava aperture (foramen) is located in the central tendon of the diaphragm at the level of T8. The inferior vena cava transmits this foramen.

2. The muscles of the thigh are divided into three groups: the anterior, medial and posterior groups. ① The anterior group consists of quadriceps femoris and sartorius. They are extensors of the knee joint and help to flex the hip joint. ② The medial group consists of pectineus, adductor longus, adductor brevis, adductor magnus and gracilis. They are chiefly adductors of the thigh. ③The posterior group consists of biceps femoris, semitendinosus and semimembranosus. They are the main extensors of the thigh and flexors of the leg. When the knee joint is flexed, they can also rotate the leg.

3. Masticatory muscles include masseter, temporalis, medial pterygoid and lateral pterygoid. The masseter, temporalis and medial pterygoid can elevate the mandible (close the mouth). Acting together, two sides of lateral pterygoids can protrude mandible and depress chin. Acting alone and alternately, they produce side-to-side movement of the mandible.

4. The sternocleidomastoid lies on the lateral side of the neck. It arises from the manubrium and upper surface of the medial one-third of the clavicle, and inserted into the mastoid process of the temporal bone. Acting alone, the head is inclined laterally and the face is rotated to the opposite side. Acting together, they thrust the head forward or raise it from pillow.

5. Biceps brachii lies on the anterior aspect of the arm. It has two heads. The short head arises from the coracoid process. The long head arises by a long narrow tendon from the supraglenoid tubercle. Two heads unite to form a flattened tendon that is inserted into the tuberosity of radius. Biceps brachii can flex elbow and shoulder joints, supinate forearm.

6. Gluteus maximus lies in the gluteal region. It arises from the dorsal portion of the iliac ala, the dorsal surface of the sacrum and coccyx, and sacrotuberous ligament. Its fibers run downward and laterally to insert into the iliotibial tract and the gluteal tuberosity of the femur. It is a powerful extensor of the thigh, the most powerful lateral rotator, and an important postural muscle.

7. It is formed by the aponeurosis of obliquus externus abdominis, obliquus internus abdominis and transversus abdominis. It has two layers. At the lateral margin of the

rectus abdominis, the aponeurosis of obliquus internus abdominis splits into two layers, the anterior layer joins with the aponeurosis of obliquus externus abdominis to form the anterior layer of the sheath and the posterior layer joins with the aponeurosis of transversus abdominis to form the posterior layer of the sheath. At the midway between the umbilicus and pubic crest, the posterior layer of the sheath forms a crescentic border, the arcuate line. Below arcuate line, the anterior layer of sheath of rectus abdominis is formed by all the aponeurosis of three flat muscles and the posterior layer of sheath is absent.

8. Quadriceps femoris lies in front surface of the thigh. It consists of four muscles. The rectus femoris arises from the anterior inferior iliac spine, the vastus medialis and vastus lateralis arise from the linea aspera, the vastus intermedius arises from the anterior surface of the femur. These four muscles unite to form a strong tendon that is inserted into the tibial tuberosity. Quadriceps femoris is the only extensor of the leg. The rectus femoris also flexes the thigh.

9. Deltoid covers the shoulder joint and forms the rounded contour of the shoulder. It arises from the lateral one-third of the clavicle, the acromion and spine of scapula. Its fibers converge to be inserted into the deltoid tuberosity of humerus. It is the most powerful abductor of the arm. Its anterior part is a strong flexor and medial rotator of the arm. The posterior part is a strong extensor and lateral rotator of the arm.

10. They are divided into two groups, the anterior group and posterior group. The anterior group consists of the superficial biceps brachii and the deep coracobrachialis and brachialis. Biceps brachii can flex the shoulder and elbow joints, supinate forearm. Coracobrachialis can flex and adduct the shoulder joint. Brachialis is the main flexor of elbow joint. The posterior group includes only one muscle, the triceps brachii. It is the chief extensor of the elbow joint. Its long head can also extend and adduct the shoulder joint.

V. Answer questions in detail

1. The shoulder joint may be abducted and adducted, flexed and extended, lateral and medial rotated. An uninterrupted succession of these movements produces circumduction.

The flexors of shoulder joint are pectoralis major, anterior part of deltoid, biceps brachii and coracobrachialis. The extensors of shoulder joint are latissimus dorsi, posterior part of deltoid, teres major and triceps brachii.

The abductors of shoulder joint are deltoid and supraspinatus. The adductors of shoulder joint are pectoralis major, latissimus dorsi, coracobrachialis, teres major and triceps brachii.

The medial rotators of shoulder joint are subscapularis, pectoralis major, latissimus dorsi, teres major and the anterior part of deltoid. The lateral rotators of shoulder joint are infraspinatus, teres minor and the posterior part of deltoid.

2. The elbow joint can do flexion, extension, pronation and supination.

   The flexors of elbow joint are biceps brachii, brachialis, brachioradialis, pronator teres, flexor carpi radialis and flexor digitorum superficialis. The extensors of elbow joint are triceps brachii and extensor digitorum.

   The pronators of elbow joint are pronator teres and pronator quadratus. The supinators of elbow joint are supinator and biceps brachii.

3. The hip joint can do flexion-extension, abduction-adduction, lateral and medial rotation, and circumduction.

   The flexors of hip joint are quadriceps femoris, iliopsoas, tensor fasciae latae and sartorius. The extensors of hip joint are gluteus maximus, biceps femoris, semitendinosus and semimembranosus.

   The adductors of hip joint are pectineus, adductor longus, adductor brevis, adductor magnus and gracilis. The abductors of hip joint are gluteus medius and gluteus minimus.

   The medial rotators of hip joint are gluteus medius and gluteus minimus. The lateral rotators of hip joint are iliopsoas, gluteus maximus, gluteus medius, gluteus minimus, piriformis, quadratus femoris, obturator internus and obturator externus.

4. The principal movements of the knee joint are flexion and extension, but the rotation is possible when this joint is in the flexed position.

   The flexors of knee joint are sartorius, biceps femoris, semitendinosus, semimembranosus, and gastrocnemius. The extensors of knee joint are quadriceps femoris.

   The medial rotators of knee joint are semitendinosus, semimembranosus and Sartorius. The lateral rotator of knee joint is biceps femoris.

Part 2   Splanchnology

Chapter 4   The General Description

Ⅰ. **Single choice**

   1. D   2. A   3. B   4. D   5. B

Ⅱ. **Double choices**

   1. AE   2. BC   3. AB   4. DE   5. DE

Chapter 5   The Alimentary System

Ⅰ. **Single choice**

1. C	2. C	3. D	4. A	5. A	6. B	7. D	8. C	9. D	10. D
11. D	12. C	13. A	14. C	15. A	16. B	17. A	18. B	19. D	20. A

21. C	22. A	23. C	24. B	25. D	26. B	27. C	28. A	29. A	30. D
31. C	32. D	33. C	34. D	35. B	36. D	37. D	38. D	39. B	40. A
41. B	42. D	43. A	44. A	45. B	46. D	47. B	48. A	49. B	50. D
51. A	52. B	53. B	54. D	55. D	56. C	57. D	58. D	59. A	60. B
61. A	62. A	63. B	64. D	65. D	66. C	67. D	68. B	69. B	70. D

Ⅱ. **Double Choices**

1. DE	2. AE	3. CD	4. BD	5. AC	6. AC	7. BD	8. BC	9. AB
10. DE	11. AC	12. AB	13. DE	14. BD	15. CE	16. CD	17. AB	18. BE
19. DE	20. CD	21. BC	22. AD	23. AE	24. BD	25. CD	26. BE	27. BC
28. DE	29. AB	30. AC						

Ⅲ. **Fill the blanks**

1. alimentary canal, digestive glands
2. parotid, sublingual gland, submandibular gland
3. pancreas
4. opposite the upper molar teeth
5. two thirds, one third
6. the palatine tonsll
7. the neck, the root, the crown
8. dentine, enamel, cement
9. periosteum covers all sockets of the alveolar processes
10. fungiform papillae, foliate papillae, filiform papillae, vallate papillae
11. apex, body, root
12. tubal torus, pharyngeal recess
13. isthmus of fauces
14. soft palatine
15. superior border of the epiglottis
16. the lower border of the cricoid cartilage
17. laryngopharynx
18. cardiac part, fundus, body, pyloric part
19. eleventh, first
20. angular incisure, intermediate groove
21. serous membrane, muscular membrane, submucosa membrane, mucous membrane
22. cardiac orifice, pyloric orifice
23. superior part, descending part, horizontal part, ascending part
24. the major duodenal papilla, the minor duodenal papilla
25. colic bands, haustra of colon, epiploic appendices
26. cecum, vermiform appendix, colon, rectum, anal canal
27. sacral flexure, perineal flexure
28. rectovesical pouch, rectouterine pouch

29. anal columns, anal valves

30. white line

31. right lobe, left lobe, quadrate lobe, caudate lobe

32. fissure for the ligamentum venosum, fissure for the ligamentum teres hepatis

33. sulcus for the inferior vena cava, fossa for the gallbladder

34. coronary ligament, right triangular ligament, left triangular ligament, falciform ligament, ligamentum teres hepatis

35. visceral surface, diaphragmatic surface

36. hepatic bare area

37. the branches of the porta vein, proper hepatic arteries, nerves to liver, hepatic ducts, lymph vessels

38. the common hepatic duct, the common bile duct

39. fundus, body, neck, cystic duct

40. head, neck, body, tail

IV. **Answer questions briefly**

1. All teeth have a similar basic structure including a crown, a root and a neck. All teeth consist of the dentine, the enamel and the cement.

2. The pharynx locates inferior to the base of skull, superior to the sixth cervical vertebra, posterior to the nose, mouth and larynx, and anterior to the cervical vertebral column.

3. The structure of the nasopharynx includes the choanae, pharyngeal opening of auditory tube, tubal torus, pharyngeal recess and pharyngeal tonsil.

4. The tonsil ring consists of lingual tonsil, palatine tonsil, tubal tonsil and pharyngeal tonsil.

5. The stomach is usually divided into four parts: the cardiac part, the fundus of stomach, the body of stomach and the pyloric of stomach.

6. The small intestine consists of the duodenum, jejunum and ileum.

7. The duodenum is divided into four parts including superior part, descending part, horizontal part and ascending part.

8. The large intestine is divided into five parts including the cecum, vermiform appendix, colon, rectum and anal canal.

9. The structure of large intestine usually is characterized by the colic bands, haustra of colon and epiploic appendices.

10. Burney's point, as the surface marking for vermiform appendix base, is the name given to the point over the right side of the abdomen that is one-third of the distance from the anterior superior iliac spine to the umbilicus (navel).

11. The key structures of anal canal include the anal columns, anal valves, anal sinus, dentate line, anal pecten and the white line.

12. According the visceral surface, the liver is divided into a right lobe, a quadrate lobe,

a left lobe and a caudate lobe.

13. The left and right hepatic duct join together to form the common hepatic duct. The common hepatic duct unites with the cystic duct to form the common bile duct.

14. The pancreas is divided into a head, neck, body and tail.

15. The gallbladder consists of the fundus, body, neck and the cystic duct.

V. Answer questions in detail

1. The pharynx is like an A-fibromuscular tube, part of digestive and respiratory systems. The pharynx extends from base of skull to the inferior border of cricoid cartilage (lower border of C_6 level);

   The pharynx is divided into three parts including the nasopharynx, the oropharynx and the laryngopharynx.

   The nasopharynx locates posterior to nasal cavities, and extends from the base of skull to level of soft palate below. The main structural features include the pharyngeal opening of auditory tube, the tubal torus and the pharyngeal recess.

   The oropharynx locates posterior to the oral cavity, below to the soft palate, and extends to upper border of epiglottis. The main structural features include the palatine tonsil lies within tonsillar fossa, the lymphatic ring consisting of pharyngeal tonsil, tonsil palatine, and lingual tonsil, forming a circular band of lymphoid tissue at oropharyngeal isthmus.

   The laryngopharynx locates posterior to larynx, and extends from upper border of epiglottis to the level of lower border of C_6. The main structural feature is the piriform recess, which is a deep depression on each side of aperture of larynx, and is the common side for lodgment of foreign bodies (for example, fish bones).

2. The stomach contains the anterior and posterior surface. It also contains the lesser curvature, which is short, concave and directed to the right and upward, near its lower part is angular incisure, and the greater curvature, which is long, convex and directed to the left and downward. At the junction of left margin of esophagus and greater curvature, stomach can be found the cardiac incisure.

   The stomach possesses the cardia and the pylorus. According to the morphology, the stomach is divided into four parts, including the cardiac part, the fundus of stomach, the body of stomach, and the pyloric part. The pyloric part also is separated into the pyloric antrum and the pyloric canal by the intermediate groove.

   The main part of stomach is situated in the left hypochondriac region, and small part can be found in the epigastric region; the cardia is situated to the left of T_{11}, and the pylorus lies to the right of L_1.

3. The liver contains the two surfaces, which are the diaphragmatic surface and the visceral surface.

   On the diaphragmatic surface, the liver is visually convex and smooth. It can be divided into right and left lobes by filiform ligament. On the visceral surface, the liver has a H-shaped fissures and grooves. These fissures and grooves are formed by the fissure for ligamentum teres hepatis and the fissure for ligamentum venosum in the left limb of H. In the right limb of H, the liver can viewed the fossa for gallbladder and the sulcus for vena cava.

The cross-bar of H is the porta hepatis, which is traversed by right and left hepatic ducts, left and right branches of proper hepatic artery and hepatic portal vein, nerves and lymphatic vessels. These structures surrounded by connective tissue is called the hepatic pedicle.

The live has the left, right, quadrate and caudate lobes. The hepatic inferior border is thin and sharp, where can be found the notch for ligamentum teres hepatis and the notch for gallbladder.

The most part of liver lies in the right hypochondriac region and epigastric region, and the less part extends into the left hypochondriac region.

4. The rectum lies within the pelvic cavity, and extends from S_3 to pelvic diaphragm. It possesses the convex backward sacral flexure and the convex forward perineal flexure in the sagittal plane.

In the coronal plane, the rectum is convex to the right in the upper and lower part and convex to the left in the middle part. In the lower part of rectum, it is dilated, which forms ampulla of rectum. There also have three transverse folds on inner surface of rectum.

Chapter 6   The Respiratory System

I . **Single choice**

1. B	2. A	3. C	4. D	5. A	6. C	7 C	8. D	9. A	10. B
11. C	12. B	13. D	14. D	15. A	6. B	17. D	18. B	19. C	20. A
21. C	22. B	23. D	24. A	25. C	26. A	27. D	28. B	29. C	30. A

II . **Double Choices**

1. BD	2. AD	3. DE	4. CE	5. AC	6. AB	7. BE	8. CD	9. AE
10. BC	11. AD	12. BE	13. AB	14. AE	15. BC	16. CE	17. DE	18. CD
19. BD	20. AC	21. AB	22. AD	23. BC	24. DE	25. CD		

III . **Fill the blanks**

1. the respiratory tract, lungs
2. Superior, middle, inferior nasal conchae
3. frontal sinus, maxillary sinus, ethmoidal sinus, sphenoidal sinus
4. sphenoethmoidal recess
5. Pharynx
6. 4 − 6 cervical
7. thyroid cartilage, cricoid cartilage, arytenoid cartilage, epiglottic cartilage
8. the aperture of larynx, the vestibular fold

9. vocal folds, cricoid cartilage

10. Carina of trachea

11. fourth thoracic vertebra, right , left principal bronchi

12. lobar bronchi, segmental bronchi, bronchioles, terminal bronchioles

13. the root of lung

14. superior, inferior lobes, oblique fissure

15. superior, middle, inferior lobes, horizontal fissure of right lung, oblique fissure

16. cardiac notch, lingual of left lung

17. diaphragmatic surface

18. parietal, visceral pleurae

19. Mediastinum

20. anterior, middle, posterior mediastinum

IV. **Answer questions briefly**

1. The trachea is located in the middle of neck and upper thorax, in front of the esopha-
    gus from the lower border of the cricoid cartilage at the level of sixth cervical vertebra
    to the level of the sternal angle. The wall of it is composed of tracheal cartilage mem-
    branous wall. It is divided into the right and left principal bronchi at inferiorly, the
    bifurcation of trachea, the carina of trachea is inside.

2. The trachea is divided into the right and left principal bronchi at the level of sternal
    angle.

    Right bronchus: 2 - 3 cm long, it is shorter, wider and more vertically. Foreign
    objects usually pass to right bronchus.

    Left bronchus: 4 - 5 cm long, it is longer, finer and less vertically.

3. Position: It is within both sides of the thorax separated from each other by the medi-
    astinum.

    Parts: The left lung is subdivided into superior and inferior lobes by an oblique
    fissure.

    The right lung is subdivided into superior, middle and inferior lobes by a hori-
    zontal fissure and an oblique fissure.

4. Parietal pleura: It lines the inner surface of chest wall and is divided into the costal
    pleura, the diaphragmatic pleura, the mediastinal pleura and the cupula of pleura (ac-
    cording to regions).

    Visceral pleura: It is on the surface of lung.

5. It is divided into superior and inferior mediastina by the line drawn horizontally from
    the sternal angle to the lower border of 4th thoracic vertebra.

    The inferior mediastinum is subdivided into an anterior mediastinum, a middle
    mediastinum, the posterior mediastinum. The middle one is occupied by the heart and
    pericardium.

V. Answer questions in detail

1. The frontal sinus: It is in the frontal bone and opens to the middle nasal meatus.

   The maxillary sinus: It is in the body of the maxilla and opens into the middle nasal meatus.

   The ethmoidal sinus: It is within the labyrinth of ethmoid bone. The anterior and middle ethmoidal sinus open into the middle nasal meatus. The posterior ethmoidal sinus drain into the superior nasal meatuses.

   The sphenoidal sinus: It is within the body of the sphenoid bone and opens into the sphenoethmoidal recess.

2. The laryngeal cavity is enclosed by the cartilages, ligaments, muscles and mucosa. There are two pairs of sagittal mucosal folds on the lateral wall of it. The upper are vestibule folds (rima vestibuli between them), the lower are vocal folds (fissure of glottis, glottis between them).

   It is divided into three parts: ①Laryngeal vestibule: from the aperture of larynx to the level of rima vestibuli. ②Intermediate cavity of larynx: between the level of rima vestibule and the fissure of glottis. ③Infraglottic cavity: from the glottis to the lower border of the cricoid cartilage.

   Ventricles of larynx: the lateral expansions of the intermediate cavity of larynx between the vestibular and the vocal folds.

3. The right lung is shorter and wider than the left one because the liver and the heart. Each lung has an apex, a base, two surfaces and three borders.

   Apex of lung is rounded and extends to about 2 - 3 cm above the level of the medial one-third of the clavicle. Base of lung is concave and related to the diaphragm, also called the diaphragmatic surface.

   Two surfaces: Costal surface is smooth, convex and related to the inner surface of the ribs, costal cartilages and intercostal spaces. Medial surface is related to the mediastinum, also called the mediastinal surface.

   Hilum of lung is a depression on the center of medial surface. The structures entering or outing hilum together form root of lung which is consists of the bronchi, pulmonary artery and vein, nerves, bronchial vessels, lymphatics and lymph nodes.

   Three borders: anterior border: thin and sharp. On the left lung has cardiac notch and lingua of left lung.

   Posterior border is round and inferior border is sharp.

Chapter 7   The Urinary System

I. Single choice

1. D	2. C	3. A	4. C	5. A	6. D	7. B	8. D	9. A	10. C
11. D	12. C	13. A	14. B	15. C	16. B	17. A	18. B	19. D	20. A
21. C	22. B	23. A	24. D	25. B	26. A	27. D	28. A	29. C	30. B

II. **Double Choices**

    1. AD   2. CE   3. AB   4. BC   5. AC   6. AE   7. CD   8. BD   9. AD

    10. DE   11. BE   12. AC   13. BD   14. BC   15. BE

III. **Fill the blanks**

1. Kidney, ureters, urinary bladder, urethra
2. fibrous capsule, adipose capsule, renal fascia
3. renal papilla
4. renal vein, renal artery, renal pelvis
5. renal artery, renal vein, renal pelvis
6. minor renal calices, major renal calices, renal pelvis
7. cortex, medulla
8. abdominal part, pelvic part, intramural part
9. two ureteric orifices, internal urethral orifice
10. apex, body, fundus, neck

IV. **Answer questions briefly**

1. According to the course, each ureter is divided into three parts.

   Abdominal part: It is continuous with the renal pelvis going downwards to the superior pelvic aperture in front of the psoas major and behind the peritoneum.

   Pelvic part: It is from superior pelvic aperture and passes downwards along the lateral wall of the lesser pelvis, then turns medially to the fundus of the urinary bladder.

   Intramural part: It passes through the wall of the urinary bladder and opens into it.

2. Three constricted areas: where urinary tract stones are likely to get stuck.

   The 1st is at the junction of the ureter and the renal pelvis. The 2nd is at the point where ureter crosses the superior aperture of the lesser pelvis. The 3rd is at the intramural part.

3. It is divided into four portions: apex, body, fundus and neck apex of bladder is toward the posterior surface of upper part of the public symphysis. Fundus of bladder is triangular shape and directed posteriorly and inferiorly. Body of bladder is situated between the apex and fundus. Neck of bladder is the lowest part of urinary bladder.

4. It is a smooth triangular area with no mucosal folds on the internal surface of the fundus of bladder, enclosed by internal urethral orifice (the anteroinferior angle) and ureteric orifices (the two posterolateral angle).

   Interureteric ridge: It is located between the two ureteric orifices as a landmark to find the ureteric orifices with cystoscope examination in the living body.

5. It is a 5 cm long narrow membranous canal that slightly curves. It extends from the bladder to external urethral orifice in the vaginal vestibule perforating the pelvic floor and urogenital diaphragm. There is urethrovaginal sphincter surrounding it.

V. Answer questions in detail

1. The kidney is a pair of bean-shaped organs. The outline of the left kidney is slender, the right one is broader and shorter. Each kidney has medial and lateral borders, anterior and posterior surfaces, superior extremity and inferior extremity.

   Superior extremity is broader and thinner than the inferior one. Anterior surface is slightly convex and posterior surface is plane. Lateral border is convex and medial border is concave, containing renal hilum, which transmits the renal vessels, nerves and a part of pelvis. The structures passing through the hilum together form the renal pedicle.

   Location: They lie on the posterior wall one on each side of the vertebral column. The right one is lower than the left. Renal hilum is at the level of 1st lumbar vertebra.

   Left kidney: superior extremity is at level of the inferior border of the body of the 11th thoracic vertebra, inferior extremity is at inferior border of the body of the 2nd lumbar vertebra.

   Right kidney: superior extremity is at level of superior border of the body of the 12th thoracic vertebra, inferior extremity is at superior border of the body of the 3rd lumbar vertebra.

2. The structures on the coronary section is divided into the cortex and medulla renal cortex: It is beneath the fibrous capsule and composed of renal glomeruli and renal tubules occupying outer 1/3 and rich in blood vessels. Renal columns is part of cortex extending inside between the pyramids.

   Renal medulla: It is deep to the cortex and composed of several renal pyramids. The base of renal pyramids is directed toward renal cortex, the apex converges towards the renal sinus and forms renal papilla. There are papillary foramina on the papilla urine through these into the lesser calices.

   Renal sinus: The minor renal calices enclose the papillae and collect urine. Major renal calyx is united by 2 - 3 minor and form the renal pelvis finally passing through the hilum and continue with the ureter. In addition, there are renal artery and its branches, renal vein and its tributaries, nerves and lymphatics, connective tissue in the renal sinus.

Chapter 8   The Reproductive System
Male Reproductive System

I. Single choice

1. D	2. D	3. C	4. D	5. D	6. D	7. B	8. A	9. C	10. C
11. C	12. C	13. D	14. A	15. C	16. B	17. C	18. A	19. C	20. A
21. C	22. B	23. C	24. D	25. A	26. A	27. C	28. B	29. C	30. D

II. Double Choices

1. AE   2. AC   3. AB   4. CD   5. AB   6. BC   7. DE   8. CD   9. AB   10. BE

III. Fill the blanks

1. prostatic portion, membranous portion, cavernous portion

2. prepubic curvature, subpubic curvature

3. ductus deferens, seminal vesicle

4. cremaster

5. prostate, seminal vesicle, bulbourethral gland

6. epididymis

7. head, body, tail

8. testicular part, funicular part, inguinal part, pelvic part

9. anterior lobe, middle lobe, posterior lobe, left lobe, right lobe

10. internal urethral orifice, membranous part, external urethral orifice

IV. Answer questions briefly

1. The internal genital organs of male reproductive system include the gonad, accessory glands and reproductive ducts. The gonad is testis; accessory glands include the prostate, the seminal vesicle and the bulbourethral gland; reproductive ducts include the epididymis, ductus deferens, ejaculatory duct and male urethra.

2. Sperm is produced in the contorted seminiferous tubules of the testis. It is stored in the epididymis through the straight seminiferous tubules, rete testis and efferent ductules of testis, and then discharged in vitro through the epididymis, ductus deferens, ejaculatory duct and urethra.

3. The spermatic cord is a soft round ropeway structure from the upper end of testis to the abdominal orifice of inguinal canal. It contains ductus deferens, testicular artery, pampiniform venous plexus, nerves and lymphatic vessels. There are three layers of coverings on the surface of spermatic cord, the external spermatic fascia, the cremaster and the internal spermatic fascia.

4. The ejaculatory duct is composed of the excretory duct of the seminal vesicle and the end of the ductus deferens. It passes through the bottom of the prostate and opens to the prostatic part of the urethra.

5. The prostate is chestnut-shaped between the urinary bladder and the urogenital diaphragm, with the pubic symphysis in the front and the rectum in the rear. The base of the prostate is adjacent to the neck of bladder, seminal vesicle and ampulla of ductus deferens, the apex is to inferior. There is a shallow sulcus along the midline of posterior surface of it. It can secret prostatic fluid, which is the main component of semen.

V. Answer questions in detail

1. The testis is located in the scrotum. There is a thick fibrous membrane on the surface of testis, called albuginea. Along the posterior margin of the testis, the albuginea

thickens and protrudes into the testis to form the testicular mediastinum. The testis is divided into several testicular lobules by connective septums that start from the mediastinum, which contain contorted seminiferous tubules, from which the sperm is produced. There are interstitial cells in the connective tissue between tubules, secreting male hormones. The contorted seminiferous tubules gradually converge to the testicular mediastinum and form the straight seminiferous tubules, then enter the testicular mediastinum and anastomose to form the testicular reticulum. The testicular efferent tubule originates from the testicular reticulum enter the epididymis passing through the posterior margin of the testis.

2. The ductus deferens arises from the tail of the epididymis and goes up to the upper part of the testis along the posterior border of the testis and inside of epididymis. It then enters the abdominal cavity passing through the inguinal canal and moves backward and downward along the lateral pelvic wall. It reaches the medial side of the seminal vesicle from the front of the ureter to the fundus of the urinary bladder, forming the ampulla of the ductus deferens. According to its course, it can be divided into testicular part (in the scrotum), spermatic part (superior to the testis), inguinal part (in the inguinal canal) and pelvic part (in pelvic cavity).

3. The male urethra originates from the internal urethral orifice of the urinary bladder and ends at the external urethral orifice of the head of penis. According to its path, it can be divided into three parts: the prostate part (through the prostate), the membranous part (through the urogenital diaphragm) and the cavernous part (through the cavernous body of urethra). It is characterized by two curvatures, three narrows and three enlargements. Two curvatures are subpubic and prepubic curvatures, three narrows are internal urethral orifice, membranous part of urethra, external urethral orifice (the most narrow), and three enlarged areas are prostatic part of urethra, bulbous part of urethra and navicular fossa of urethra.

Female Reproductive System

Ⅰ. **Single choice**

1. A   2. A   3. D   4. B   5. C   6. B   7. D   8. A   9. D   10. A

11. C   12. C   13. D   14. B   15. C   16. D   17. B   18. D   19. B   20. C

21. A   22. D   23. D   24. D   25. A   26. D   27. D   28. B   29. C   30. D

Ⅱ. **Double Choices**

1. AE   2. AB   3. AC   4. AC   5. DE   6. AC   7. BC   8. BD   9. AD   10. AD

Ⅲ. **Fill the blanks**

1. internal, external

2. suspensory ligament of ovary, proper ligament of ovary

3. uterine part, isthmus of uterine tube, ampulla of uterine tube, infundibulum of uterine tube

4. vulva

5. uterine orifice, abdominal orifice

6. fundus, body, isthmus, cervix

7. suspensory ligament

8. cavity of uterus, canal of cervix of uterus

9. broad ligament of uterus, round ligament of uterus, cardinal ligament of uterus, uterosacral ligament of uterus

10. greater vestibular gland

IV. **Answer questions briefly**

1. The internal genital organs of female reproductive system include the gonad, accessory glands and reproductive ducts. The gonad is ovary; accessory gland includes the greater vestibular glands; reproductive ducts include the uterine tube, uterus and vagina.

2. The ovary is located in the ovarian fossa of the lateral pelvic wall at the angle between the internal and external iliac arteries. It is oblate and oval shaped, divided into upper and lower ends, medial and lateral surfaces, anterior and posterior borders. The upper end is fixed to the pelvic wall by the suspensory ligament of ovary (with ovarian blood vessels), and the lower end is connected to the fundus of the uterus by the proper ligament of ovary.

3. The uterine tube can be divided into uterine part, isthmus, ampulla and infundibulum, four parts from medial to lateral. The isthmus of uterine tube is narrow and short, which is the clinical site for tubal ligation. The ampulla of uterine tube is broad and long, which is the fertilized part of ovum.

4. The internal cavity of uterus is divided into the cavity of uterus and canal of cervix. The cavity of uterus is a triangular space, surrounded by the body and fundus of the uterus, which connects with the uterine orifice of the uterine tube; the apex of cavity of uterus is down to the canal of cervix. The canal of cervix is spindle-shaped, located in the cervix, the upper orifice is called the internal orifice of uterus, and the lower orifice is called the external orifice of uterus.

5. The upper part of vagina surrounds the vaginal part of cervix of uterus. The annular depression between them is called vaginal fornix, which can be divided into anterior, posterior and bilateral parts. The posterior vaginal fornix is the deepest part. There are only the posterior vaginal wall and peritoneum between the posterior vaginal fornix and the rectouterine pouch. Puncture of peritoneal cavity can be performed clinically through this area.

V. **Answer questions in detail**

1. The uterine tubes are a pair of curved trumpet-shaped muscular ducts. They connect to both sides of fundus of uterus and lie in upper part of broad ligament of uterus. The whole length of it can be divided into four parts: uterine part, isthmus of uterine

tube, ampulla of uterine tube and infundibulum of uterine tube from medial to lateral. The isthmus of uterine tube is narrow and short, which is the surgical site for tubal ligation in clinic. The ampulla of uterine tube is broad and long, which is the fertilized part of ovum. The uterine tube has two orifices: the uterine orifice and the abdominal orifice, which are opened in the uterine cavity and the peritoneal cavity respectively.

2. The uterus is a slightly flat inverted pear-shaped organ. According to the shape, it can be divided into the fundus, body, isthmus and cervix four parts. The fundus of uterus is the part above the uterine orifice of the uterine tubes on both sides, the middle part is the body of uterus, and the lower part is the cylindrical cervix. The lower part of the cervix goes into the vagina, so the cervix can be divided into the supravaginal part and the vaginal part of cervix. The narrow area at the junction of uterine body and cervix is isthmus of uterus.

   The internal cavity of uterus is divided into the cavity of uterus and canal of cervix. The cavity of uterus is a triangular space and surrounded by the body and fundus of the uterus, which connects to the uterine orifice of the uterine tube; the apex of cavity of uterus is down to the canal of cervix. The canal of cervix is spindle-shaped, located in the cervix, the upper orifice is called the internal orifice of uterus, and the lower orifice is called the external orifice of uterus.

3. The uterus is located in the center of the lesser pelvis, between the urinary bladder and rectum, and above the vagina, showing a slight anteversion and anteflexion. Anteversion refers to the whole uterus tilting forward and forming an angle of about 90 degrees with the vagina; anteflexion is formed between the body of the uterus and the cervix, about 170 degrees.

   The location of uterus depends mainly on the support of muscles of pelvic floor and the pulling of ligaments. The broad ligament of the uterus, a frontal double-layer peritoneal formation, connecting the uterus to the lateral wall of the lesser pelvis, is to maintain the median position of the uterus. The round ligament of the uterus, originating from the fundus of the uterus and passing through the inguinal canal to the subcutaneous tissue of the greater lip of pudendum, is to maintain the anteversion of the uterus. The cardinal ligament of the uterus, which connects the cervix to the lateral wall of the pelvis, can maintain the uterus in the pelvis and prevent from uterine prolapse. The uterosacral ligament, originating from the back of the cervix and inserting at the front of the sacrum around both sides of the rectum, pulls the uterus backward and upward, and maintains the anteversion and anteflexion of the uterus.

Chapter 9   The Peritoneum and the Perineum

Ⅰ. Single choice

   1. C   2. A   3. D   4. B   5. A   6. B   7. D   8. C   9. B   10. C

11. C   12. A   13. C   14. B   15. D   16. A   17. C   18. C   19. A   20. D

II. **Double Choices**

1. BD   2. BD   3. AE   4. AE   5. BD

III. **Fill the blanks**

1. intraperitoneal organ
2. intraperitoneal organ
3. extraperitoneal organ
4. greater omentum, lesser omentum
5. hepatogastric ligament, hepatoduodenal ligament
6. proper hepatic artery, common bile duct, hepatic portal vein
7. jejunum and ileum, vermiform appendix, transverse colon, sigmoid colon
8. uterovesical pouch, uterorectal pouch
9. urogenital triangle, anal triangle
10. urethra, vagina

IV. **Answer questions briefly**

1. The peritoneal cavity is a sac formed by the continuation of the visceral peritoneum and the parietal peritoneum. In male it is closed, while in the female it opens to the outside of body by the reproductive duct. About the peritoneal fossae in the pelvic cavity, there are rectovesical pouch in male and vesicouterine and rectouterine pouches in female. Rectouterine pouch is the lowest point of the peritoneal cavity.

2. The main structures formed by the peritoneum include the omentum (greater and lesser omenta), the mesentery (mesentery of small intestine, mesoappendix, transverse mesocolon and sigmoid mesocolon), the ligaments (falciform ligament and coronal ligament of liver, splencogastric ligament, etc.), and pouches (rectovesical pouch in male, vesicouterine and rectouterine pouches in female).

3. The lesser omentum is a bilayer peritoneum connecting the hilum of the liver to the lesser curvature of the stomach and the upper part of the duodenum. It can be divided into left hepatogastric ligament and right hepatoduodenal ligament. The common bile duct (right anterior), the proper hepatic artery (left anterior) and the hepatic portal vein (posterior) course in hepatoduodenal ligament.

4. There are falciform ligament, right and left coronal ligament, right and left triangular ligament, hepatogastric ligament, hepatoduodenal ligament

5. The urogenital diaphragm is composed of the supradiaphragmatic fascia, the infradiaphragmatic fascia, the deep transverse perineal muscle and the sphincter urethrae. In male the urethra passes through it, while in female the urethra and vagina passes.
The pelvic diaphragm is composed of the superior pelvic fascia, the inferior pelvic fascia and the levator ani and coccygeus between them, with the anal canal passing through.

V. **Answer questions in detail**

1. According to whether the surface of organ covering by peritoneum, there are three

types:

First, the intraperitoneal organ: all surface of the organ covered by the peritoneum is intraperitoneal organ, such as stomach, jejunum, spleen, etc.

Second, the intraperitoneal organ: most of the surface of organ covered by the peritoneum is intraperitoneal organ, such as liver, ascending colon, uterus, etc.

Third, the extraperitoneal organ: only one surface of the organ covered by the peritoneum is extraperitoneal organ, such as kidney, pancreas, etc.

2. The perineum has a broad and narrow sense of perineum. Generalized perineum refers to all soft tissues that closing the pelvic outlet. The narrow sense of perineum refers to the soft tissue between the anus and the external genitals. Generally, the perineum is diamond-shaped. Its anterior border is the lower edge of pubic symphysis, the posterior border is the tip of coccyx, and its bilateral boundary is the inferior pubic ramus, ischial ramus, ischial tuberosity and sacrotuberous ligament. The line that is between the both ischial tuberosities divides the perineum into the anterior urogenital region and the posterior anal region. The former has urethra in male, while the urethra and vagina in female; the latter has anal canal in both.

Part 3   The Circulatory System

Chapter 10   The General Description and the Heart

I. **Single choice**

   1. A   2. B   3. D   4. C   5. B   6. D   7. B   8. D   9. D   10. A

11. C   12. A   13. D   14. C   15. D   16. B   17. B   18. B   19. D   20. C

21. D   22. B   23. D   24. A   25. B   26. B   27. D   28. C   29. A   30. A

31. C   32. C   33. D   34. B   35. C

II. **Double Choices**

  1. AB   2. AC   3. BD   4. CD   5. BC   6. BD   7. BE   8. AD   9. CE   10. BC

III. **Fill the blanks**

  1. cardiovascular system, lymphatic system

  2. greater (systemic), lesser (pulmonary)

  3. artery, vein, capillary

  4. atrium proper, sinus venarum cavarum

  5. anterior interventricular groove, posterior interventricular groove

  6. anterior interventricular branch, great cardiac

  7. annulus of tricuspid valve, tricuspid valve, tendinous cord, papillary muscle

  8. supraventricular crest

  9. anterior cusp of the bicuspid valve

   10. left coronary artery, right coronary artery

   11. orifice of the inferior vena cava, orifice of the superior vena cava, orifice of the coro-
       nary sinus

   12. fibrous pericardium, serous pericardium

   13. parietal layer of the serous pericardium, visceral layer of the serous pericardium

   14. sinoatrial node

   15. right bundle branch

Ⅳ. **Answer questions briefly**

   1. The cardiovascular system comprises the heart, arteries, capillaries and veins. The
      heart is the "pump" of the circulation, distributing the blood to all parts of the body.
      Arteries are vessels that carry the blood away from the heart. The veins are vessels
      that transport the blood from capillary networks to the heart. The capillaries are ves-
      sel networks that connect the terminal arteries with terminal veins.

   2. The passage of the blood through the heart and blood vessels constitute what is
      termed as the blood circulation. The course of the blood from the left ventricle
      through the body generally to the right atrium of the heart constitutes the greater cir-
      culation or systemic circulation, while the passage from the right ventricle through
      the lungs to the left atrium of the heart is termed the lesser circulation or pulmonary
      circulation.

   3. The conduction system of the heart includes sinoatrial node, atrioventricular node,
      the atrioventricular bundle with its left and right branches and the subendocardial
      plexus of Purkinje fibers.

   4. The arteries of the heart are right and left coronary arteries. The right coronary ar-
      tery arises from the right aortic sinus. Its main branches are the posterior interven-
      tricular branch, the posterior branch of the left ventricle, the right conus artery and
      so on. The left coronary artery arises from the left aortic sinus and its main branches
      are the anterior interventricular branch, circumflex branch, etc.

   5. Coronary sinus collects the great cardiac vein, the middle cardiac vein and the small
      cardiac vein, then along the coronary groove opens into the right atrium. In addition,
      there are anterior cardiac veins and smallest cardiac veins.

Ⅴ. **Answer questions in detail**

   1. The heart lies in the middle mediastinum posterior to the sternum and costal cartila-
      ges and rests on the superior surface of the diaphragm. The heart assumes an oblique
      position, 2/3 lies on left side of the midline and 1/3 on right side.

      The heart is conically shaped with its apex formed by left ventricle pointing to-
      wards to the left, anteriorly and inferiorly of the midline. The heart's base is quadri-
      lateral formed by atria and faces backward, upward and to the right.

      Two surfaces: the surfaces of the heart may be divided into anterior or sterno-
      costal surface and inferior or diaphragmatic one.

Three borders: the right border is formed by right atrium mainly, left border is formed by left ventricle mainly and inferior border is formed by right and left ventricles. There is an apical notch in inferior border just right to the apex.

Four grooves: coronary groove separating atria and ventricles, anterior and posterior interventricular grooves separating both ventricles, interatrial groove separating both atria behind. There is the atrioventricular crux at the junction area of posterior interventricular groove and coronary groove.

2. The right atrium has two parts: a posterior part (sinus venarum cavarum) and an anterior part (atrium proper). These two parts of the atrium are separated by the crista terminalis or sulcus terminalis. In the atrium proper there are pectinate muscle. The anterior, extending part of the atrium proper is called right auricle. On the right side of the interatrial septum, there are fossa ovalis and triangle of Koch.

The right atrium have three entrances: the superior vena cava and inferior vena cava and the coronary sinus to receive blood. The right atrium opens into the right ventricle through the right atrioventricular orifice.

3. The right ventricle has two parts: sinus part (inflow tract) and infundibular part (outflow tract). These two parts of the right ventricle are separated by supraventricular crest.

In the inflow tract, there are trabeculae carneae. The right atrioventricular orifice is the inlet of the right ventricle. Tricuspid complex includes the annulus of the tricuspid, the tricuspid valve (anterior, posterior and medial cusps), the tendinous cords and the papillary muscles. The septomarginal trabecula or moderate band extends from the interventricular septum to the base of the anterior papillary muscle.

The outflow tract has the conus arteriosus, pulmonary orifice, and pulmonary valve (anterior, left and right cusps). The semilunar valves are constructed to permit the flow of blood in only one direction.

Chapter 11   The Arteries

I. **Single choice**

1. A   2. D   3. C   4. D   5. A   6. B   7. B   8. A   9. B   10. D
11. D   12. D   13. B   14. C   15. A   16. C   17. A   18. B   19. C   20. B
21. B   22. C   23. C   24. A   25. A

II. **Double Choices**

1. AD   2. DE   3. BC   4. AC   5. BE   6. CE   7. AB   8. CE   9. CE
10. CE   11. BD   12. AC   13. BE   14. BC   15. DE

III. **Fill the blanks**

1. ascending aorta, aortic arch, descending aorta
2. brachiocephalic trunk, left common carotid artery, left subclavian artery
3. right common carotid artery, right subclavian artery

4. carotid sinus

5. carotid body

6. superficial temporal artery, maxillary artery

7. terminal branch of the ulnar artery, superficial palmar branch of the radial artery

8. celiac trunk, superior mesenteric artery, inferior mesenteric artery

9. middle suprarenal artery, renal artery, testicular artery or ovarian artery

10. superior thyroid artery, inferior thyroid artery

11. inferior phrenic artery, renal artery

12. celiac trunk, proper hepatic artery

13. splenic artery, gastroduodenal artery

14. common hepatic artery, left gastric artery, splenic artery

15. medial malleolus

Ⅳ. **Answer questions briefly**

1. The axillary artery is the continuation of the subclavian artery. It begins at the outer border of the first rib and ends at the lower border of the teres major where it becomes the brachial artery. Its chief branches are thoracoacromial artery, lateral thoracic artery, subscapular artery, anterior circumflex humeral artery and posterior circumflex humeral artery.

2. The superficial palmar arch is covered by the palmar aponeurosis, and lies on the flexor tendons of the fingers. Its convexity is placed at the level of a line drawn across the hand from the distal border of the root of the extended thumb. It is formed mainly by the superficial palmar branch of the radial artery and the terminal branch of the ulnar artery.

3. There are three pairs of arteries on the suprarenal glands. The first is the superior suprarenal artery that comes from the inferior phrenic artery. The second is the middle suprarenal artery that comes from the abdominal aorta. The last is the inferior suprarenal artery that arises from the renal artery.

Ⅴ. **Answer questions in detail**

1. There are at least five arteries supplying blood to the stomach. Those arteries form anastomoses along the lesser curvature and the greater curvature. The left gastric artery arises from the celiac trunk and runs along the lesser curvature of the stomach to the pylorus. The right gastric artery arises from the proper hepatic artery, descends in the right part of lesser omentum to the pylorus, passes left along the lesser curvature and ends by anastomoses with the left gastric artery.

   The short gastric artery, starts from the splenic artery along the greater curvature to the fundus of stomach, supplying it with blood. The left gastroepiploic artery comes from the splenic artery then goes right along the greater curvature. The right gastroepiploic artery comes from the gastroduodenal artery and goes left along the greater curvature. They form anastomoses along the greater curvature. In addition, there is a posterior gastric artery supplying blood to the stomach from splenic artery.

2. The aorta leaves the heart, goes superiorly and arcs to left side, and then descends along the bodies of the vertebrae to the inferior part of the abdomen. According to this course, the aorta is divided into the following three parts.

The ascending aorta arises from the left ventricle and ascends for only about 5 cm. It lies posterior to the pulmonary trunk, passes to the right of it and curves left to become the aortic arch.

The aortic arch arches posteriorly and to the left, the aortic arch lies posterior to the manubrium of the sternum.

The descending aorta is continuing from the aortic arch at level of T_4 vertebral body, the descending aorta runs downward posterior to the heart and inferiorly in frontal of the vertebral column. It has two parts, the thoracic aorta and the abdominal aorta. The thoracic aorta descends on the bodies of the thoracic vertebrae just to the left of the midline. The thoracic aorta passes through the aortic hiatus of diaphragm at the level of vertebra T_{12} and enters the abdominal cavity as the abdominal aorta, which lies on the lumbar vertebral bodies in the midline. The abdominal aorta ends at the level of vertebra L_4, where it divides into the right and left common iliac arteries.

Chapter 12　The Veins

Ⅰ. **Single choice**

    1. D   2. A   3. C   4. A   5. A   6. B   7. C   8. B   9. D   10. C

    11. D   12. A   13. B   14. D   15. D   16. D   17. B   18. A   19. C   20. B

    21. C   22. D   23. B   24. C   25. C

Ⅱ. **Double Choices**

    1. CE   2. BD   3. AB   4. AE   5. AC   6. AD   7. CD   8. CE   9. BC   10. AC

Ⅲ. **Fill the blanks**

    1. external jugular vein

    2. cephalic vein, basilic vein, median cubital vein

    3. superficial lateral femoral vein, superficial medial femoral vein, superficial iliac circumflex vein, superficial epigastric vein, external pudendal vein

    4. sinus of dura mater, diploic vein

    5. inferior vena cava, left renal vein

    6. popliteal vein

    7. cephalic vein, basilic vein

    8. inferior vena cava, left renal vein

    9. abdominal aorta, sulcus of the inferior vena cava

    10. occipital vein, posterior auricular vein, posterior division of retromandibular vein

Ⅳ. **Answer questions briefly**

1. The characteristics of veins include larger cavity, thinner wall, lower pressure and slower flow than their arterial counterparts. The systemic veins can be divided into superficial veins and the deep veins. The deep veins usually accompany the coursing arteries. Most veins are provided with the valves in the inner surface of the wall. Lastly, there are numerous anastomoses among the veins.

2. The dangerous area is located at the region of the facial vein around the nose and the upper lip. The facial vein has no valves above the angle of the month, and it communicates with the cavernous sinus by angular vein and superior ophthalmic vein. Thus, the infective factor of the face may enter facial vein and then into the intracranial venous sinuses, lead to infection in cavernous sinus.

3. The inferior vena cava is the largest venous trunk, formed by the junction of the two common iliac veins at the anterior of the fifth lumbar vertebra. It ascends along the right side of the abdominal aorta, and then passes the sulcus for the inferior vena cava of liver and the vena cava foramen of the diaphragm, in the end it joins into the right atrium.

Ⅴ. **Answer questions in detail**

1. The great saphenous vein begins from the dorsal venous arch of the foot at the medial margin of the foot, passes in front of the medial malleolus and ascends to the knee along the medial side of the leg. It runs upwards posteromedial to the medial condyle of the femur, along the medial side of the thigh, then to the front of the thigh. It perforates the saphenous hiatus at about 3 – 4 cm of the inferior of the pubic tubercle and drains into the femoral vein.

   The important tributaries of the great saphenous vein are the superficial lateral femoral vein, the superficial medial femoral vein, the external pudendal vein, the superficial iliac circumflex vein and the superficial epigastric vein.

2. The hepatic portal vein is a short trunk, it collects the blood from the unpaired organs in the abdominal cavity and the rectum in the pelvic cavity. The hepatic portal vein and its tributaries send the blood from those organs to the liver.

   Its tributaries include superior mesenteric, splenic, inferior mesenteric, left gastric, right gastric, cystic and paraumbilical veins. The superior mesenteric vein receives the blood from the organs supplied by the superior mesenteric artery and gastroduodenal artery. The splenic vein collects the blood from the organs supplied by the splenic artery. The inferior mesenteric vein runs in accompany with the corresponding artery and opens into the splenic vein or the superior mesenteric vein or opens into the union of the two. The left and right gastric veins collect blood from the lesser curvature of the stomach. The cystic vein collects blood from the wall of the gallbladder. The paraumbilical veins run along the ligamentum teres, and then open into the left branch of the hepatic portal vein.

The main anastomoses between the hepatic portal venous system and vena cava system are as follows:

(1) Anastomoses through the esophageal venous plexus: hepatic portal vein—left gastric vein—esophageal vein—azygos vein—superior vena cava.

(2) Anastomoses through the rectal venous plexus: hepatic portal vein—splenic vein—inferior mesenteric vein—superior rectal vein—rectal venous plexus—inferior rectal or anal veins—internal iliac vein—common iliac vein—inferior vena cava.

(3) Anastomoses through the periumbilical venous plexus:

hepatic portal vein—paraumbilical vein—periumbilical venous rete—thoracoepigastric or superior epigastric veins—lateral thoracic or internal thoracic veins—finally to superior vena cava.

hepatic portal vein—paraumbilical vein—periumbilical venous rete—superficial epigastric or inferior epigastric veins—external iliac vein—finally to inferior vena cava.

Chapter 13   The Lymphatic System

Ⅰ. **Single choice**

   1. C   2. A   3. D   4. A   5. B   6. D   7. B   8. D   9. A   10. C

  11. D 12. C 13. A 14. D 15. A 16. C 17. B 18. D 19. B 20. A

Ⅱ. **Double Choices**

   1. AE 2. AC 3. BD 4. AB 5. AE 6. AB 7. DE 8. BD 9. BE 10. BE

Ⅲ. **Fill the blanks**

1. lymph conducting channels, lymphoid tissues, lymphoid organs
2. diffused lymphoid tissues, lymph nodules
3. right jugular trunk, right subclavian trunk, right bronchomediastinal trunk
4. right lumbar trunk, left lumbar trunk, intestinal trunk
5. intestinal trunk
6. left venous angle
7. spleen
8. lymphatic capillary, lymphatic vessel, lymphatic trunk, lymphatic duct
9. hilum of lymph node
10. cubital lymph node

Ⅳ. **Answer questions briefly**

1. The lymphatic system is an accessory system of the cardiovascular system. It consists of the lymph conducting channels, lymphatic tissues and lymphoid organs. The lymph conducting channels include the lymphatic capillaries, lymphatic vessels, lymphatic trunks and lymphatic ducts. The lymphatic tissues consist of the diffused lymphoid tissues and the lymph nodules. The lymphoid organs include lymph nodes, tonsils, thymus and spleen.

2. There are nine lymphatic trunks, 4 pairs and 1 single, in human body. The paired trunks are right and left jugular trunks, the right and left subclavian trunks, the right and left bronchomediastinal trunks, the right and left lumbar trunks. The single one is the intestinal trunk.

3. The lymph nodes are small, oval or bean-shaped bodies. The color of the lymph node is usually grayish pink. Generally, each has a hilum on one side, through which the blood vessels and nerves enter or leave the node. The efferent lymphatic vessel also emerges from the node at the hilum. The afferent lymphatic vessels enter lymph nodes in different parts of the periphery.

4. The axillary lymph nodes are in the loose connective tissues of the axillary fossa and are arranged along the blood vessels. They are divided into 5 groups: anterior group or pectoral lymph nodes, lateral lymph nodes, posterior or subscapular lymph nodes, central lymph nodes and apical lymph nodes.

V. Answer questions in detail

1. The thoracic duct is the left lymphatic duct and markedly longer than the right lymphatic duct. Its most inferior part, located at the union of the right and left lumbar and intestinal trunks, is the cisterna chyli which lies on the bodies of vertebrae L_1 and L_2. From there, the thoracic duct ascends along the vertebral bodies. In the superior thorax, it turns left and empties into the venous circulation at the left venous angle. The thoracic duct is often joined by the left jugular, subclavian, and/or bronchomediastinal trunks just before it joins with the venous circulation. The thoracic duct drains three-quarters of the body: the left side of the head, neck, and thorax; the left upper limb; and the body's entire lower half.

2. Efferent vessels of the mammary gland mainly drain to the axillary lymph nodes. There are three drainage directions:

    (1) Efferent vessels of the lateral and central parts drain to the pectoral lymph nodes;

    (2) Efferent vessels of the superior part to the apical lymph nodes and supraclavicular nodes;

    (3) Efferent vessels of the medial part to the parasternal lymph nodes.

    Superficial lymphatic vessels of the medial part communicate with the opposite side. The lymphatic vessels of the mediainferior part communicate with the hepatic lymphatic vessels by the epigastric lymphatic vessels and inferior phrenic lymphatic vessels.

Part 4   The Sensory System

Chapter14   The Visual Organs

Ⅰ. **Single choice**

   1. A   2. D   3. B   4. B   5. B   6. A   7. C   8. C   9. B   10. D

   11. D   12. C   13. B   14. C   15. A   16. B   17. A   18. C   19. D   20. A

   21. B   22. D   23. D   24. B   25. C   26. B   27. A   28. A   29. D   30. C

Ⅱ. **Double Choices**

   1. BD   2. BD   3. CD   4. BE   5. BE   6. AC   7. BD   8. CE   9. BE

   10. BE   11. AE   12. DE   13. DE   14. AB   15. AD

Ⅲ. **Fill the blanks**

   1. fibrous tunic; vascular tunic; inner tunic

   2. cornea; sclera

   3. iris; ciliary body; choroid

   4. ciliary body

   5. aqueous humor; lens; vitreous body

   6. optic part; ciliary part; iridial part

   7. iridial part; ciliary part

   8. bipolar cell; ganglion cell

   9. cornea; aqueous humor; lens; vitreous body

   10. chambers of eye

   11. optic disc

   12. fovea centralis

   13. cornea

   14. iris

   15. superior rectus; lateral rectus; medial rectus; inferior rectus; superior obliquus; inferior obliquus; levator palpebrae superioris

Ⅳ. **Answer questions briefly**

   1. The structures of the eyeball that with refractive effect include cornea, aqueous humor, lens and vitreous body. The cornea is the anterior one-sixth portion of the fibrous tunic. It is colorless and transparent, but with abundant nerve innervations. The aqueous humor fills the chamber of eye. The lens is located between iris and vitreous body. The vitreous body is located in the posterior portion of the eyeball.

   2. The retina is the inner tunic of the eyeball. It can be divided into three portions from back forwards: optic part, ciliary part and iridial part. Near the center of the posterior part of the retina, there is macula lutea with the highest visual acuity. About

3.5 cm to the nasal side of the macula lutea, there is a site where optic nerve fibers piercing and leaving the retina, which has no photoreceptor cell and is insensitive to light, thus referred to as the blind spot.

3. The vascular tunic consists of three portions: from the front backwards, they are iris, ciliary body and choroid. The iris is located at the anterior portion of the vascular tunic. At the center of the iris, there is a foramen called pupil, which is the only passage for light to enter the eyeball. The diameter of the pupil changes with the intensity of the light. The contraction of the dilator pupillae can enlarge the pupil, whereas the contraction of sphincter pupillae can constrict the pupil. The ciliary body has the function of secreting aqueous humor and adjusting of the diopter of the lens. The choroid is abundant in blood vessels, which has the function of offering nutrition for the eyeball.

4. The eyelid includes five layers. They are skin, subcutaneous alveolar tissue, orbicularis oculi, tarsus and conjunctiva.

5. The extraocular muscles include superior rectus, lateral rectus, medial rectus, inferior rectus, superior obliquus, inferior obliquus, levator palpebrae superioris.

Ⅴ. Answer questions in detail

1. The extraocular muscles include superior rectus, lateral rectus, medial rectus, inferior rectus, superior obliquus, inferior obliquus and levator palpebrae superioris. The lateral rectus is innervated by abducent nerve. Levator palpebrae superioris is attached to the upper eyelid and the other muscles are all attached to eyeball. The superior obliquus is innervated by trochlear nerve. And the other muscles are all innervated by oculomotor nerve.

2. The three tunics of the eyeball include fibrous tunic, vascular tunic and inner tunic. The fibrous tunic is the outer layer and consists of cornea and sclera. Cornea is the anterior one-sixth portion of the fibrous tunic. It is colorless and abundant in nerve innervations. The vascular tunic consists of three portions: from the front backwards, they are iris, ciliary body and choroid. The iris is located at the anterior portion of the vascular tunic. At the center of the iris, there is a foramen called as pupil, which is the only passage for light entering the eyeball. The diameter of the pupil can change with the intensity of the light. The contraction of the dilator pupillae can enlarge the pupil, whereas the contraction of sphincter pupillae can constrict the pupil. The ciliary body has the function of secreting aqueous humor and adjusting of the diopter of the lens. The choroid is abundant in blood vessels, which has the function of offering nutrition for the eyeball. The retina is the inner tunic of the eyeball. It can be divided into three portions from back forwards; they are optic part, ciliary part and iridial part. Near the center of the posterior part of the retina, there is macula lutea with the highest visual acuity. About 3.5 cm to nasal side of the macula lutea, there is a site where optic nerve fibers piercing and leaving the retina, which has no

photoreceptor cell and is insensitive to light and is referred to blind spot.

3. The contents of the eyeball include aqueous humor, lens and vitreous body. Aqueous humor fills the chamber of the eyeball, which has the functions of offering nutrition for the cornea and helping to maintain the intraocular pressure. The lens is a colorless structure lacking vessels and nerves and is located between iris and vitreous body. The lens has very important refractive effect on the light and helps to focus a clear image of the object on the retina. The vitreous body is located in the posterior portion of the eyeball and offers important supporting function on the retina.

Chapter 15　The Vestibulocochlear Organ

Ⅰ. **Single choice**

1. B　　2. C　　3. C　　4. D　　5. B　　6. A　　7. C　　8. D　　9. D　　10. A

11. C　　12. A　　13. A　　14. B　　15. B　　16. B　　17. D　　18. D　　19. A　　20. D

21. D　　22. B　　23. C　　24. D　　25. B

Ⅱ. **Double Choices**

1. BE　　2. CE　　3. CE　　4. AD　　5. BE　　6. AC　　7. DE　　8. AE　　9. CE

10. BC　　11. CD　　12. DE　　13. AE　　14. CD　　15. CD

Ⅲ. **Fill the blanks**

1. external ear; middle ear; inner ear

2. sound; movement

3. mastoid antrum; tympani cavity; auditory tube

4. second tympanic membrane

5. bony semicircular canals; vestibule; cochlea

6. anterior semicircular canal; lateral semicircular canal; posterior semicircular canal

7. macula utriculi; macula sacculi

8. utricle; saccule

9. promontory; fenestra vestibuli; fenestra cochlea; prominence of facial canal

10. endolymph

11. perilymph

12. basilar membrane

13. base of the stapes, annular ligament

14. auditory tube

15. superior wall (tegmental wall); lateral wall (membranous wall); medial wall (labyrinthine wall); inferior wall (jugular wall); posterior wall (mastoid wall); anterior wall (carotid wall)

Ⅳ. **Answer questions briefly**

1. The external acoustic meatus extends from the external acoustic pore to the tympanic membrane. It is about 2.1 – 2.5 cm in length. The external meatus has two parts: the lateral cartilaginous part and medial bony part. The cartilaginous part accounts

for 1/3 of the total length of the meatus; the bony part accounts for 2/3 of the total length of the meatus. The external acoustic meatus is not a straight canal; it is a curved structure. In clinical examination for adult, in order to expose the tympanic membrane, drawing the auricle upwards is necessary.

2. The six walls of the tympanic cavity are superior wall, lateral wall, medial wall, inferior wall, posterior wall and anterior wall. The superior wall is a thin plate of compact bone referred to tegmen tympani. So the superior wall is also called as tegmental wall. The lateral wall is almost entirely formed by the tympanic membrane. So the lateral wall is also called as membranous wall. The medial wall is formed by the lateral wall of the bony labyrinth, so it is also called as labyrinthine wall. The inferior wall is adjacent to the internal jugular vein and also called as jugular wall. The posterior wall is communicating with the mastoid antrum and called as mastoid wall. The anterior wall is adjacent to internal carotid artery and called as carotid wall.

3. The middle ear is made of tympanic cavity, mastoid antrum, mastoid cells and auditory tube. The tympanic cavity is located in the middle portion of the middle ear. It has six walls: superior wall, lateral wall, medial wall, inferior wall, posterior wall and anterior wall. It communicates with the mastoid antrum and mastoid cells through the opening of the mastoid antrum posteriorly and with the nasopharynx through auditory tube anteriorly. Inside the tympanic cavity, there are three auditory ossicles: malleus, incus and stapes.

4. The bony labyrinth consists of three parts. They are bony semicircular canals, vestibule and cochlea. We have three bony semicircular canals: anterior semicircular canal, posterior semicircular canal and lateral semicircular canal. These semicircular canals are located in the posterior portion of the whole bony labyrinth. The cochlea is a conical structure resembling snail and is composed of cochlear spiral canal, modiolus and osseous spiral lamina. The cochlea is located in the anterior portion of the whole bony labyrinth. The vestibule is located between the bony semicircular canals and the cochlea.

5. The membranous labyrinth is composed of membranous semicircular ducts, utricle, saccule and cochlear ducts. The membranous semicircular ducts are located inside the bony semicircular canals. Inside the ampulla of the membranous semicircular ducts, there are ampullary crests, which is responsible for the receiving of the rotation movement information. Utricle and saccule are located inside the vestibule and possessing macula utriculi and macula sacculi respectively, which are responsible for the collecting of the linear acceleration or deceleration movement information. The cochlear duct is situated in the cochlear spiral canals. In the basilar membrane of the cochlear duct, there are spiral organs which are responsible for the collecting the auditory sensation.

Ⅴ. **Answer questions in detail**

1. The six walls of the tympanic cavity are superior wall, lateral wall, medial wall, inferior wall, posterior wall and anterior wall. The superior wall is a thin plate of compact bone referred to tegmen tympani. So the superior wall is also called as tegmental wall. The lateral wall is almost entirely formed by the tympanic membrane. So the lateral wall is also called as membranous wall. The medial wall is formed by the lateral wall of the bony labyrinth, so it is also called as labyrinthine wall. The inferior wall is adjacent to the internal jugular vein and also called as jugular wall. The posterior wall is communicating with the mastoid antrum and called as mastoid wall. The anterior wall is adjacent to internal carotid artery and called as carotid wall. The tympanic cavity communicates with the mastoid antrum and mastoid cells through the opening of the mastoid antrum posteriorly and with the nasopharynx through auditory tube anteriorly. Inside the tympanic cavity, there are three auditory ossicles: malleus, incus and stapes.

2. The labyrinth is composed of bony labyrinth and membranous labyrinth.

   The bony labyrinth consists of three parts. They are bony semicircular canals, vestibule and cochlea. We have three bony semicircular canals: anterior semicircular canal, posterior semicircular canal and lateral semicircular canal. These semicircular canals are located in the posterior portion of the whole bony labyrinth. The cochlea is a conical structure resembling snail and is composed of cochlear spiral canal, modiolus and osseous spiral lamina. The cochlea is located in the anterior portion of the whole bony labyrinth. The vestibule is located between the bony semicircular canals and the cochlea.

   The membranous labyrinth is composed of membranous semicircular ducts, utricle, saccule and cochlear ducts. The membranous semicircular ducts are located inside the bony semicircular canals. Inside the ampulla of the membranous semicircular ducts, there are ampullary crests, which is responsible for the receiving of the rotation movement information. Utricle and saccule are located inside the vestibule and possessing macula utriculi and macula sacculi respectively, which are responsible for the collecting of the linear acceleration or deceleration movement information. The cochlear duct is situated in the cochlear spiral canals. In the basilar membrane of the cochlear duct, there are spiral organs which is responsible for the collecting the auditory sensation.

3. The sound wave — external acoustic meatus — tympanic membrane — chain of the auditory ossicles — fenestra vestibule — perilymph within the scala vestibule — helicotrema — perilymph within the scala tympani — endolymph within the cochlear duct — spiral organs — nerve impulse.

Part 5　The Nervous System

Chapter 16　The Spinal Cord

Ⅰ. **Single choice**

1. D	2. C	3. D	4. C	5. C	6. C	7. A	8. C	9. D	10. C
11. A	12. B	13. A	14. C	15. D	16. C	17. A	18. A	19. B	20. B
21. C	22. A	23. A	24. B	25. B	26. A	27. D	28. D	29. D	30. C
31. D	32. D	33. A	34. D	35. D					

Ⅱ. **Double Choices**

1. AB　2. AD　3. CD　4. AC　5. CD　6. AB　7. AB　8. BC　9. AB　10. DE

Ⅲ. **Fill the blanks**

1. brain, spinal cord
2. neuron, neuroglia
3. astrocyte, oligodendrocytes, microglia
4. cervical enlargement, lumbosacral enlargement
5. conus medullaris
6. filum terminale
7. whiter matter, grey matter
8. Central canal
9. anterior funiculus, lateral funiculus, posterior funiculus
10. fasciculus gracilis, fasciculus cuneatus
11. αmotor neuron, γmotor neuron, Renshaw cell
12. anterior white commissure
13. grey commissure
14. C_4, T_1
15. L_1, S_3
16. nucleus proprius
17. cerebral cortex, internal capsule, brain stem
18. convey impulse, reflex
19. nucleus
20. ganglion

Ⅳ. **Answer questions briefly**

1. Anatomically, it contains the central nervous system(CNS) and peripheral nervous system(PNS), the CNS has the brain and spinal cord and PNS consists of cranial and spinal nerves. Functionally, it is divided into somatic nervous system and autonomic nervous system, which innervates the structure of body wall and activities of the vis-

ceral organs respectively.

2. Reflexes are subconscious stimulus-response mechanism. The reflex arc includes the receptor, afferent neurons, interneuron, efferent neurons and effector. The effector can produce the response.

3. Nerve cells with the common shape, function and connections within the CNS are grouped together into nucleus. Nerve cells with the common shape, function and connections outside the CNS are grouped together into ganglion.

4. It contains the long ascending tracts: fasciculus gracilis, fasciculus cuneatus, posterior spinocerebellar tract, anterior spinocerebellar tract, spinothalamic tract; the long descending tracts, including the corticospinal tract, tectospinal tract, rubrospinal tract, vestibulospinal tract and reticulospinal tract.

5. The nuclei in the posterior horn contain the nucleus posteromarginalis, the substantia gelatinosa, the nucleus proprius and the nucleus thoracicus.

6. The long descending tracts in the white matter are concerned with somatic movement, visceral innervation and the modification of muscle tone, they mostly arise from the cerebral cortex or brain stem, they are the corticospinal tract, the tectospinal tract, the rubrospinal tract, the vestibulospinal tract and the reticulospinal tract.

7. The long ascending tracts contain the fasciculus gracilis, fasciculus cuneatus, posterior spinocerebellar tract, anterior spinocerebellar tract, spinothalamic tract.

8. One of the principal function of the spinal cord is to convey afferent impulses, which initiates from the somatic and visceral receptors to the brain and to conduct efferent impulse from the brain to the effectors. A second principal function is related to the reflexes, it plays the part of the center of the segmental reflex arc.

V. **Answer questions in detail**

1. The spinal cord, a long cylindrical structure, is located in the vertebral canal and invested by meninges. It extends from the foramen magnum, where itconnects with the medulla oblongata, to the lower border of the first lumbar vertebra, about 40－45 cm in length. Diameters of the spinal cord are not equal at different levels, as there are two enlargements: the cervical and the lumbosacral enlargements. Caudal to the lumbosacral enlargement, the spinal cord tapers gradually and becomes the conical termination known as conus medullaris. A condensation of pia mater forms the filum terminale that descends from the conus medullaris to the level of the 2nd sacral vertebra, from here it is enveloped by the dura mater and continues to the posterior surface of the coccyx.

   A longitudinal fissure and some sulci are shown on the surface of the naked spinal cord. They are the anterior median fissure, posterior median sulcus, posterolateral sulci and anterolateral sulci.

   The spinal cord has 31 external segments, each segment is functionally correlated with the related cutaneous area, skeletal muscles and viscera.

2. The corticospinal tract arises from the cerebral cortex, descends through the internal capsule and brain stem. It can be divided into two tracts:

The lateral corticospinal tract decussates in the medulla oblongata and descends medially to the posterior spinocerebellar tract in the spinal cord. The tract extends to the most caudal part of the spinal cord and progressively diminishes in size as more and more fibers leave to terminate in the anterior horn of the grey matter. The tract has somatotopical arrangements from medial to lateral in cervical, thoracic, lumbar and sacral order. The anterior corticospinal tract occupies a strip adjacent to the anterior median fissure and normally extends only to the upper thoracic spinal segments. Most of the fibers decussate in the anterior commissure before they terminate in the anterior horn.

Both tracts give rise to the motor fibers that leave the spinal cord through the anterior roots to be distributed by way of spinal nerves to skeletal muscles.

Chapter 17   The Brain Stem

Ⅰ. **Single choice**

1. D   2. A   3. D   4. A   5. B   6. D   7. B   8. A   9. C   10. D
11. C   12. B   13. C   14. A   15. D   16. D   17. C   18. C   19. B   20. D
21. B   22. C   23. A   24. C   25. D   26. C   27. D   28. A   29. C   30. D

Ⅱ. **Double Choices**

1. DE   2. AB   3. AB   4. AC   5. AE   6. BE   7. DE   8. CD   9. BE   10. AB

Ⅲ. **Fill the blanks**

1. medulla oblongata, pons, midbrain
2. gracile tubercle, cuneate tubercle
3. basilar sulcus
4. abducent nerve, facial nerve, vestibulocochlear nerve
5. sulcus limitans, median sulcus
6. striae medullares
7. genu of facial nerve, abducent nucleus
8. hypoglossal triangle, vagal triangle
9. cerebral peduncles, interpeduncular fossa
10. superior colliculus , inferior colliculus
11. motor nucleus of trigeminal nerve
12. glossopharyngeal, vagus, accessory
13. accessory oculomotor nucleus, superior salivatory nucleus, inferior salivatory nucleus, dorsal nucleus of vagus nerve
14. vestibular nucleus, cochlear nucleus
15. internal arcuate fibers
16. substantia nigra

17. anterior spinothalamic tract, lateral spinothalamic tract

18. tegmentum, crus cerebri

19. trigeminal lemniscus

20. inferior cerebellar peduncle

Ⅳ. **Answer questions briefly**

1. Medial lemniscus arises from the fibers of internal arcuate fibers, which are efferent fibers emerging from the gracile and cuneate nuclei. It terminates at the ventral posterolateral nucleus of thalamus. The medial lemniscus is an important tract for conducting proprioceptive and fine touch sensations of the contralateral trunk and limbs.

2. The boundaries of the rhomboid fossa:

   Superior border: superior cerebellar peduncles, superior medullary velum Inferior border: the inferior cerebellar peduncles, and the cuneate and gracile tubercles

   The external features of the rhomboid fossa: the rhomboid fossa is divided into symmetrical halves by median sulcus, lateral to median sulcus is medial eminence. The medial eminence is bounded laterally by sulcus limitans. Striae medullares divide the rhomboid fossa into pontine and medullary parts. Superior fovea is adjacent to the top of the sulcus limitans. Locus ceruleus is deep to the fovea. At the middle of the medial eminence above the striae medullares, a rounded swelling is facial colliculus. Below the striae medullares on each side of the median sulcus, there are two triangular areas. The medial one is hypoglossal triangle. The lateral one is vagal triangle. Vestibular area is a triangular area lateral to the sulcus limitans.

3. Nucleus of oculomotor nerve, trochlear nerve, abducent nerve, give off nerves to innervate the extraocular muscles, the fibers innervate the sphincter pupillae and ciliary muscle arise from the accessory nucleus of oculomotor nerve in brain stem.

4. The nucleus of facial nerve gives off the special visceral efferent fibers, supplying the muscles of expression. The superior salivatory nucleus gives off the general visceral efferent fibers relayed in parasympathetic ganglia. The postganglionic fibers are distributed to the lacrimal gland, the submandibular and sublingual glands. The nucleus of solitary tract receives the afferent fibers related to the taste sensation of the anterior two-thirds of tongue.

5. Nucleus of hypoglossal nerve lies under the hypoglossal triangle. It gives off fibers to form the hypoglossal nerve to innervate muscles of tongue.

   Spinal and pontine nuclei of trigeminal nerve receive the impulse of general somatic sensation from the anterior two-thirds of the tongue through trigeminal nerve.

   Nucleus of solitary tract receive the impulses of general visceral sensation from the posterior one-third of tongue, as well as taste impulses from the tongue.

6. In brain stem, outside the more conspicuous fiber bundles and nuclei, there is an extensive field of intermingled grey and white matter collectively termed the reticular formation.

The fibers contributing to the reticular formation interlace each other to form wide-spread network. The neurons contributing to the reticular formation can make up nuclei. The reticular formation is an important integration center for the vital activity. Its main functions include the somatomotor control, activation of the behavioral arousal, visceromotor control, etc.

7. The ventral surface of the midbrain is a pair of cerebral peduncles. A deep depression bounded by the cerebral peduncles is known as interpeduncular fossa. The oculomotor nerve emerges from the medial side of the peduncle. On the dorsal surface of the midbrain, there are four rounded eminences, the superior and inferior colliculi (corpora quadrigemina, quadrigeminal body). From lateral aspect of each colliculus, there is a brachium. The brachium of superior colliculus passes inferiorly to the lateral geniculate body. The brachium of inferior colliculus ascends to the medial geniculate body.

8. There are eight nuclei in the brain stem are related to the movement of skeletal muscles in head and neck. Nuclei of oculomotor, trochlear and abducent nerves innervate the movement of extraocular muscles. Nucleus of hypoglossal nerve innervate the muscles of tongue. Motor nucleus of trigeminal nerve innervates masticatory muscles. Nucleus of facial nerve innervates expression muscles. Nucleus ambiguous gives off fibers to join the glossopharyngeal, vagus and accessory nerves respectively, and supply the muscles of pharynx and larynx. Nucleus of accessory nerve innervate the sternocleidomastoid and trapezius.

V. Answer questions in detail

1. On the dorsum of the section is the lower part of fourth ventricle. A median sulcus and a pair of sulcus limitans are appeared on the rhomboid fossa. The nucleus of hypoglossal nerve, dorsal nucleus of vagus nerve and vestibular nuclei are situated in the gray matter of the floor of fourth ventricle from medial to lateral. Inferior cerebellar peduncle is ventrolateral to the vestibular nuclei.

   On the ventral side of the section, the olive with the inferior olivary nuclei are located lateral to the pyramid. The pyramidal tracts are located in the pyramids. Closely dorsal to the pyramidal tracts are the medial lemniscus, tectospinal tract and medial longitudinal fasciculus from ventral to dorsal. The rootlets of the hypoglossal nerve traverse between the pyramidal tract and the inferior olivary nucleus and emerge from the surface of the medulla oblongata to constitute the hypoglossal nerve.

2. The trapezoid body intermingles with the medial lemniscus and separates the basilar part from the tegmentum of pons. Pontine nuclei are located in the basilar part of the pons. The transverse fibers arise from the pontine nuclei are collected as the pontocerebellar fibers, which continue transversely to become middle cerebellar peduncle. The longitudinal bundles of fibers in the basilar part are pyramidal tract and corticopontine tract.

In the tegmentum, the nucleus of abducent nerve and the internal genu of facial nerve underlie the facial colliculus. Lateral to the sulcus limitans are the vestibular nucleus and, more deeply, the spinal nucleus and tract of trigeminal nerve. The nucleus of facial nerve is situated at the ventrolateral part of the reticular formation, ventromedial to the spinal tract and nucleus of trigeminal nerve.

3. The canal in this section is the cerebral aqueduct. The periaqueductal grey matter is around the canal. The nucleus of trochlear nerve is situated on its ventromedial part, the mesencephalic nucleus of trigeminal nerve is on its lateral margin. Dorsolaterally to the central grey matter are a pair of nuclei of inferior colliculi. The substantia nigra separates the tegmentum from the crus cerebri. Crus cerebri is formed by the pyramidal tract in the middle 3/5, frontopontine tract in the medial 1/5 and parito-occipito-temporo-pontine tracts in lateral 1/5. The tegmentum is formed by the reticular formation mainly. The medial, trigeminal and spinal lemnisci are in the ventrolateral portion of the tegmentum.

Chapter 18   The Cerebellum

I. **Single choice**

1. A   2. B   3. A   4. A   5. D   6. A   7. C   8. B   9. D   10. D

11. B   12. D   13. A   14. D   15. D

II. **Double choices**

1. DE   2. AB   3. DE   4. BD   5. AE

III. **Fill the blanks**

1. hemispheres vermis

2. the superior cerebellar peduncle the middle cerebellar peduncle the inferior cerebellar peduncle

3. the flocculonodular lobe the anterior lobe the posterior lobe

4. the fastigial nucleus the globose nucleus the emboliform nucleus the dentate nucleus

5. the molecular layer the Purkinje layer the granular layer

IV. **Answer questions briefly**

1. The cerebellum is occupies the posterior cranial fossa. It is posterior to the medulla and pons and inferior to the occipital lobes of the cerebrum. The cerebellum is shaped like a butterfly. The central constricted area is called the vermis, and lateral lobes are referred to as hemispheres.

2. The projection fibers of cerebellum connect the cerebellum with other parts of the brain and the spinal cord. They are grouped into three peduncles on each side: the inferior cerebellar peduncle (restiform body), the middle cerebellar peduncle (brachium pontis) and the superior cerebellar peduncle (brachium conjunctivum)

3. The surface of the cerebellum, called the cortex, consists of gray matter. The cerebellar cortex uniformly structured in all parts and divided into three layers, they are

the molecular layer, the Purkinje cell layer and the granular layer. The only fibers leaving the cortex are axons of Purkinje cells.

Ⅴ. **Answer questions in detail**

1. Four pairs of nuclei are embedded deeply in the medullary center; they are the fastigial, globose, emboliform and dentate nuclei. The fastigial nucleus receives the fibers from the archicerebellum; the globose and emboliform nuclei receive most fibers from the spinocerebellum; the dentate nucleus receives the fibers from the pontocerebellum.

2. The cerebellum can be divided into three portions; the flocculonodular lobe (vestibulocerebellum or archicerebellum), the anterior lobe and the rostral part of the inferior vermis are also called the spinocerebellum or paleocerebellum and the the posterior lobe (pontocerebellum or neocerebellum). The main function of the flocculonodular lobe is related to maintaining equilibrium and controlling posture; the main function of the spinocerebellum is concerned with adjusting muscular tonicity; the posterior lobe functions in coordinating movements of the body's skeletal muscles.

Chapter 19   The Diencephalon

Ⅰ. **Single choice**

1. A	2. D	3. A	4. C	5. B	6. D	7. C	8. B	9. C	10. B
11. A	12. D	13. A	14. A	15. D	16. B	17. A	18. C	19. C	20. B

Ⅱ. **Double choices**

1. BD   2. AC   3. BD   4. BD   5. AC

Ⅲ. **Fill the blanks**

1. the dorsal thalamus, the hypothalamus, the epithalamus, the subthalamus, the metathalamus

2. the anterior nuclear group, the medial nuclear group , the posterior nuclear group

3. the reticular nucleus, the midline and intralaminar nuclei, the specific thalamic nuclei, the nonspecific thalamic nuclei

4. the lateral geniculate body, the medial geniculate body

5. the pineal body, the right and left habenular trigone (nuclei) , the habenular commissure, the posterior commissure

6. the lamina terminalis, the optic tracts, the optic chiasma, the mammillary body, tuber cinereum, the infundibulum, the hypophysis

Ⅳ. **Answer questions briefly**

1. The thalamic masses are, by the internal medullary lamina, divided into an anterior nuclear group, a medial nuclear group, and a lateral nuclear group. The lateral nuclear group consists of ventral tier (the medial and lateral geniculate nuclei, the ventral posterior, ventral lateral and ventral anterior nuclei) and dorsal tier (the pulvinar, lateral posterior nuclei and lateral dorsal nuclei).

2. The diencephalon is located between the brain stem and the hemispheres of the cere-brum, being almost entirely surrounded by the hemispheres of the cerebrum, only the ventral surface of the diencephalon can be viewed. It consists of the dorsal thalamus, hypothalamus, epithalamus, subthalamus, and metathalamus.

3. The metathalamus is located posterolaterally to the thalamus. It includes lateral ge-niculate body and medial geniculate body. The lateral geniculate nucleus is located in lateral geniculate body and then gives rise to the optic radiation. In medial geniculate body the medial geniculate body is located, the medial geniculate body then gives rise to the acoustic radiation.

Ⅴ. **Answer questions in detail**

The specific thalamic nuclei comprise the ventral tier of the lateral nuclear mass and send fibers to sensory and motor areas of cortex. The medial nucleus (hearing), lateral genic-ulate nucleus (vision), and the ventral posterior nucleus (general sensations) are special sensory nuclei. The ventral posterior nucleus consists of the ventral posteromedial nucle-us(receiving fibers from the trigeminal lemniscus) and the ventral posterolateral nucleus (receiving fibers from the medial lemniscus and spinothalamic lemniscus). The ventral lateral and ventral anterior nuclei are special motor nuclei.

Chapter 20   The Telencephalon

Ⅰ. **Single choice**

  1. A   2. B   3. B   4. D   5. D   6. A   7. D   8. C   9. B   10. C

  11. C   12. C   13. A   14. C   15. B   16. C   17. C   18. B   19. A   20. B

  21. C   22. A   23. A   24. B   25. C   26. B   27. C   28. D   29. A   30. C

Ⅱ. **Double Choices**

  1. AC   2. AB   3. AD   4. CD   5. AD   6. AC   7. BC   8. AC   9. DE   10. AD

Ⅲ. **Fill the blanks**

  1. cerebral longitudinal fissure, cerebral transverse fissure

  2. frontal lobe, parietal lobe, temporal lobe, occipital lobe, insular lobe

  3. precentral gyrus, superior frontal gyrus, middle frontal gyrus, inferior gyrus

  4. hippocampus, dentate gyrus

  5. caudate nucleus, lentiform nucleus, claustrum, amygdaloid body

  6. putamen, globus pallidus, globus pallidus

  7. body, anterior horn, posterior horn, inferior horn, interventricular foramen

  8. transverse temporal gyrus, calcarine sulcus

  9. inferior frontal gyrus, motor aphasia

  10. angular gyrus, alexia

  11. association fibers, commissural fibers, projection fibers

  12. rostrum, genu, trunk and splenium

  13. superior longitudinal fasciculus, inferior longitudinal fasciculus, uncinate fasciculus,

cingulum

14. anterior limb, genu, posterior limb

15. central thalamic radiation, optic radiation, acoustic radiation

IV. Answer questions briefly

1. In the temporal lobe, the superior and inferior temporal sulci divide the lateral surface of the temporal lobe into superior, middle and inferior temporal gyri. The upper surface of the superior temporal gyrus forms the floor of the lateral sulcus and presents two transverse temporal gyri.

2. In the frontal lobe, the precentral sulcus is in front of and parallel to the central sulcus, these sulci outline the precentral gyrus. The remaining surface of the frontal lobe is divided into superior, middle and inferior gyri by superior and inferior frontal sulci, which are roughly perpendicular to the precentral sulcus.

3. They connect the gyri in one hemisphere to the gyri in the other hemisphere, most of these fibers constitute the corpus callosum, the remainder are included in two very small bundles, the anterior and posterior commissures. The corpus callosum can be divided into 4 parts: the rostrum, genu, body and splenium from forward backward.

4. It is located in the precentral gyrus, including the anterior wall of the central sulcus and the anterior part of the paracentral lobule on the media surface of the hemisphere. The motor cortex is 4.5 mm in thickness, in which giant pyramidal cells of Betz are present in the fifth layer. The main sources to this area are premotor cortex, the somesthetic cortex and the ventral lateral and ventral anterior thalamic nuclei.

5. The limbic system usually includes the limbic lobe as well as associated subcortical structures, such as the amygdaloid complex, hypothalamus. epithalamus, anterior thalamic nuclei. It extends even more to include the medial tegmental region of the midbrain and the raphe nuclei of the brain stem.

6. Broca's area or the motor speech area occupies the opercular and triangular portion of the inferior frontal gyrus. corresponding with areas 44 and 45 of Brodmann. The posterior portion of the middle frontal gyrus is the written word area. The auditory speech and visual speech areas are situation the posterior part of the temporal gyri and the inferior parietal lobule.

7. They are several masses of gray matter situated in the central portion of the cerebral hemisphere, including corpus striatum, claustrum and the amygdaloid. The corpus striatum has the caudate nucleus and the lentiform nucleus.

V. Answer questions in detail

1. The internal capsule consists of an anterior limb, a genu and a posterior limb, which have topographic relationships with adjacent grey masses. The anterior limb is bounded by the lenticular nucleus and the head of the caudate nucleus, and the genu is medial to the apex of the lentiform nucleus. The posterior limb includes the following parts: The thalamolentiform part is between the lentiform nucleus and the thala-

mus; the retrolentiform part consists of fibers occupying the region behind the lentiform nucleus, ans the sublentiform part includes those fibers that pass through the posterior part of the lentiform nucleus.

The anterior thalamic radiation, which is included in the anterior limb of the internal capsule, consists mainly of fibers connecting the dorsomedial thalamic nucleus and the prefrontal cortex. The middle thalamic radiation is a component of the posterior limb of the internal capsule, includes the projection from the ventral posterior thalamic nucleus to the somesthetic area in the parietal lobe. The posterior thalamic radiation contained in the retrolentiform part establishes connections between the thalamus and cortex of the occipital lobe. The optic radiation ending in the visual cortex and the acoustic radiation, which originates in the medial geniculate nucleus and terminates in the acoustic area.

2. They are roughly C-shaped cavities lined by ependymal epithelium one in each cerebral hemisphere, and filled with the CSF. Each lateral ventricle consists of a body on the region of the parietal lobe from which anterior, posterior and inferior horns extend into the frontal, occipital and temporal lobes, respectively. The lateral ventricle communicates with the third ventricle through the interventricular foramen. The body of the lateral ventricle, situated mainly in the parietal lobe, has a flat roof formed by the corpus callosum, its floor includes part of the dorsal surface of the thalamus. The anterior horn extends forward in the frontal lobe and the inferior horn includes a particularly important structure, the hippocampus.

Portion of the ventricle contains choroid plexus, formed by an invagination of pia matter covering layer of ependymal on the medial surface of the cerebral hemisphere.

Chapter 21   The Nervous Pathways

Ⅰ. **Single choice**

1. A	2. B	3. D	4. D	5. D	6. C	7. A	8. D	9. C	10. A
11. C	12. B	13. C	14. B	15. B	16. C	17. B	18. A	19. B	20. A
21. D	22. C	23. D	24. D	25. A	26. B	27. C	28. B	29. A	30. B

Ⅱ. **Double Choices**

1. AD   2. BC   3. AB   4. BE   5. AC   6. AB   7. DE   8. AE   9. CE   10. AC

Ⅲ. **Fill the blanks**

1. corticospinal tract, corticonuclear tract
2. medial lemniscus, spinothalamic tract
3. spinal ganglion, lamina Ⅰ, Ⅳ to Ⅶ of spinal cord, ventroposterolateral nucleus of thalamus
4. spinal ganglion, gracile and cuneate nuclei, ventroposterolateral nucleus of thalamus
5. medial lemniscus, spinothalamic tract, trigeminal lemniscus
6. bipolar cells, ganglion cells, lateral geniculate body

7. the fibers come from ipsilateral temporal retina, the fibers come from contralateral nasal retina

8. trigeminal lemniscus, posterior limb of internal capsule, inferior part of postcentral gyrus

9. central radiation of thalamus, posterior limb of internal capsule, middle and upper part of postcentral gyrus, posterior part of paracentral lobule

10. corticonuclear tract

11. the precentral gyrus, the anterior part paracentral lobule

12. central thalamic radiation, corticospinal tract, optic radiation, acoustic radiation

13. trigeminal ganglion, spinal nucleus of trigeminal nerve, pontine nucleus of trigeminal nerve

14. corticospinal tract, corticonuclear tract

15. spinothalamic tract

IV. **Answer questions briefly**

1. Rod and cone cell—bipolar cell—Ganglionic cell—optic nerve—optic chiasma—nasal fibers of retina—optic tract—lateral geniculate nucleus—optic radiation—posterior limb of the internal capsule   both banks of calcarine sulcus.

2. Optic nerve—optic tract—brachium of superior colliculus—pretectal area—bilaterally E-W nucleus (accessory nucleus of oculomotor nerve)—ciliary ganglion—sphincter of the iris.

3. Trigeminal ganglia — spinal and pontine nucleus of trigeminal nerve — goes to opposite side — upward and forms trigeminal lemniscus — runs up — ventroposteromedial nucleus of thalamus—central thalamic radiation—posterior limb of the internal capsule—inferior part of the postcentral gyrus.

4. The upper motor neurons are the giant pyramidal cells and other pyramidal cells with various sizes, which are located in the precentral gyrus and anterior part of paracentral lobule. Their axons form the descending pyramidal tract, among which, the fibers ending in the cranial motor nuclei are called the corticonuclear tract and those terminating in the anterior horn of the spinal cord are called corticospinal tract.

5. Extrapyramidal system comprise cerebral cortex, striate body, dorsal thalamus, subthalamus, tectum of the midbrain, red nucleus, substantia nigra, pontine nuclei, vestibular nuclei, cerebellum, reticular formation of brain stem and their fibers.

   The functions of extrapyramidal system are regulating the tonicity of the muscles, coordinating the muscular activities, maintaining the normal body posture and producing habitual and rhythmic movements.

V. **Answer questions in detail**

1. The superficial sensory pathway of trunk and limb is concerned with pain and thermal sensations:

   Skin (exteroceptor) — peripheral process — (pseudounipolar).

spinal ganglia — lateral bundle — spinal cord — synapse with the cells — I ,
IV-VII — run upward one or two segments and cross through the anterior white commissure — reach the opposite lateral funiculus — to form lateral and anterior spinothalamic tract — spinal lemniscus — runs up — ventroposterolateral nucleus of
thalamus — central thalamic radiation — posterior limb of the internal capsule — superior and middle parts of the postcentral gyrus, and the posteror part of the paracentral lobule.

2. Muscle, tendon, joint, skin — spinal ganglia — medial bundle — posterior funiculus
   — fasciculus gracilis and fasciculus cuneatus — gracile and cuneate nuclei — cross
   through the central canal — reach the opposite side — upward named medial lemnisci
   — runs up — ventroposterolateral nucleus of thalamus — central thalamic radiation
   — posterior limb of the internal capsule — superior and middle parts of the postcentral gyrus, the paracentral lobule, and precentral gyrus.

3. Superior and middle parts of the precentral gyrus, and the anterior part of the paracentral lobule upper motor neurons — corticospinal tract — pass through posterior
   limb of internal capsule — crus cerebral base, the basilar part of the pons and pyramid of medulla oblongata — pyramidal decussation — lateral corticospinal tract —
   uncross — anterior corticospinal tract the motor neurons of the anterior horn — lower
   motor neurons — skeletal muscles.

Chapter 22   The Meninges and Blood Vessels and the Cerebrospinal Fluid

I . **Single choice**

1. C	2. B	3. A	4. B	5. D	6. C	7. C	8. A	9. C	10. C
11. D	12. D	13. B	14. C	15. D	16. D	17. D	18. D	19. C	20. D
21. B	22. D	23. D	24. A	25. C	26. C	27. D	28. D	29. A	30. C

II . **Double choices**

1. AD   2. BE   3. AB   4. AC   5. CE   6DE   7. AE   8. CE   9. AE   10. DE

III . **Fill the blanks**

1. cerebral dura mater; cerebral arachnoid mater; cerebral pia mater
2. arachnoid granulations
3. Tentorium of cerebellum
4. blood-brain barrier; blood-CSF barrier; CSF-brain barrier
5. Internal carotid artery; abducent nerve
6. interventricular foramina; cerebral aqueduct
7. sinuses of dura mater
8. vertebral artery; internal carotid artery
9. cerebral falx; cerebellar falx
10. tentorial incisures
11. anterior cerebral artery; middle cerebral artery; anterior choroid artery; posterior

communicating artery

12. anterior cerebral artery; posterior cerebral artery; anterior communicating artery; posterior communicating artery; internal carotid artery

13. cortical; central

14. endothelial cells, astrocyte end-feet; capillary basement membrane

15. lenticulostriate

IV. Answer questions briefly

1. Arising from the common carotid artery on each side of the head and neck, the internal carotid runs vertically upward in the carotid sheath and enters the skull through the carotid canal to enter the cranial cavity. Then, the artery passes through the internal wall of the cavernous sinus to the brain.

2. The left and right internal carotid arteries arise from the left and right common carotid arteries. The left and right anterior cerebral arteries arise from the left and right internal carotid arteries. The posterior communicating artery is given off as a branch of the internal carotid artery. The right and left posterior cerebral arteries arise from the basilar artery. The anterior communicating artery arises from either the left or right side of anterior cerebral arteries.

3. From lateral ventricle, CSF passes through the interventricular foramina to the third ventricle, then the cerebral aqueduct to the fourth ventricle. The fluid passes into the subarachnoid space from the openings of fourth ventricle: the median foramen and the two lateral foramina. Then, CSF goes into the cerebral veins via the arachnoid granulations.

4. The tentorium of cerebellum partially separates the cerebellum and brainstem from the cerebrum. The cerebral falx partially separates the two hemispheres of the brain. The cerebellar falx partially separates the cerebellar hemispheres. The sellar diaphragm forms a partial roof over the hypophysial fossa.

5. The sinuses of dura mater are venous channels between the endosteal and meningeal layers of dura mater in the brain. The walls of the dural sinuses are composed of dura mater lined with endothelium. They lack a full set of veins, e. g. smooth muscle and valves. Consequently, the sinuses can be injured by head trauma and the bleeding of the sinuses is much difficult to stop.

6. The internal carotid artery and abducent nerve run through the inter wall of the sinus. The oculomotor, trochlear, ophthalmic and maxillary divisions of the trigeminal nerve pass through its lateral wall.

7. The blood of the spinal cord comes from the anterior, posterior spinal arteries of the vertebral artery, and from the posterior intercostal arteries and the lumbar arteries.

V. Answer questions in detail

1. (1) Anterior cerebral artery is a pair of arteries on the brain that supplies most midline portions of the frontal lobes and superior medial parietal lobes.

Cortical branches: supply a part of the frontal lobe, specifically its medial surface and the upper border. They also supply the front four-fifths of the corpus callosum.

Central branches: anterior limb of the internal capsule, anterior part of the caudate nucleus and lentiform nucleus.

(2) Middle cerebral artery.

Cortical branches: the bulk of the lateral surface of the hemisphere and insular lobe, including the somatic motor area, somatic sensory area and language center.

Central branches: supply the caudate nucleus and lentiform nucleus as well as the genu and posterior limb of internal capsule.

(3) Anterior choroid artery: supplies choroid plexus of the lateral ventricle and third ventricle, lateral geniculate body, posterior limb of internal capsule, globus pallidus and hippocampus, et al.

(4) Posterior communicating artery: connects the internal carotid arteries and posterior cerebral arteries. This provides redundancies or collaterals in the cerebral circulation.

2. Cerebrospinal fluid (CSF) is a clear, colorless body fluid found in the brain and spinal cord. It is produced by the specialised ependymal cells in the choroid plexuses of the ventricles of the brain. There is about 125 mL of CSF at any one time, and about 500 mL is generated every day.

CSF occupies the subarachnoid space and the ventricular system around and inside the brain and spinal cord. It fills the ventricles of the brain, cisterns, and sulci, as well as the central canal of the spinal cord.

CSF is produced by the choroid plexuses of the lateral, the third and the fourth ventricles. From lateral ventricle, CSF passes through the interventricular foramina to the third ventricle, then the cerebral aqueduct to the fourth ventricle. The fluid passes into the subarachnoid space from the openings of fourth ventricle: the median foramen and the two lateral foramina. CSF moves in a single outward direction from the ventricles, but multidirectionally in the subarachnoid space. From subarachnoid space, CSF is absorbed by the arachnoid granulations and then drained into the sinuses of dura mater and cerebral veins.

3. Spinal dura mater is a thick membrane made of dense irregular connective tissue that surrounds the spinal cord. It is the outermost of the three layers of membrane of the spinal cord. Laterally, the spinal dura is continuous with the external membrane of the spinal nerve at the intervertebral foramina. The spinal epidural space is the space between the dura and the periosteum of the vertebral canal. In humans, the epidural space contains lymphatics, spinal nerve roots, loose connective tissue, fatty tissue, small arteries, and a network of internal vertebral venous plexuses. The space is not

open into the cranial cavity.

Spinal arachnoid is a delicate, avascular membrane lying between the dura and pia mater. The spinal arachnoid is separated from the pia mater by the subarachnoid space containing the cerebrospinal fluid. Spinal subarachnoid space is continuous with cerebral arachnoid space. The spinal subarachnoid space becomes wider from the inferior end of the spinal cord to about the level of the second sacral vertebra, which is called terminal cistern and contains the cauda equina.

Spinal pia mater is the delicate innermost layer of the membranes surrounding the spinal cord. 21 pairs of denticulate ligaments, which composed of spinal pia mater, help to anchor the spinal cord to the dura mater. At the end of the spinal cord, the membrane extends as a thin filament called the filum terminale, which attaches to the back of the coccyx.

Because spinal nerves on each side pass through the epidural space, this space is applicable for block anesthesia, called epidural anesthesia. Because the spinal subarachnoid space is continuous with cerebral arachnoid space, and there is no spinal cord in the terminal cistern, the terminal cistern is the best site for a lumbar puncture to collect cerebrospinal fluid, with which many diagnoses may be supported or excluded. Injuries involving the meninges can result in a subarachnoid hemorrhage, epidural hematoma or subdural hematoma.

Chapter 23   The Spinal Nerves

I. **Single choice**

1. B 2. A 3. C 4. D 5. D 6. C 7. C 8. B 9. C 10. D
11. A 12. B 13. B 14. C 15. C 16. D 17. D 18. A 19. B 20. B
21. C 22. B 23. D 24. A 25. A 26. D 27. B 28. C 29. B 30. B
31. A 32. B 33. A 34. D 35. B

II. **Double Choices**

1. BC 2. AE 3. AD 4. CD 5. AE 6. CE 7. AC 8. BE 9. BD
10. DE 11. AD 12. AB 13. CD 14. DE 15. BC

III. **Fill the blanks**

1. somatic sensory, somatic motor, visceral sensory, visceral motor
2. anterior, posterior, meningeal, communicating
3. lesser occipital nerve, great auricular nerve, transverse nerve of neck, supraclavicular nerve
4. the 4 lower cervical (C_{5-8}) and great part of the anterior branch of the 1st thoracic nerve (T_1)
5. biceps brachii, brachialis, coracobrachialis, musculocutaneous
6. radial, ulnar, median
7. median, ulnar

8. sternal angle, umbilicus

9. inferior gluteal, pudendal, posterior femoral cutaneous

10. tibial

11. semimembranosus, semitendinosus, biceps femoris, sciatic

12. iliohypogastric, ilioinguinal, lateral femoral cutaneous, femoral

13. the anterior branches of the 5th, a part of the 4th lumbar nerve

14. medial sural cutaneous nerve, tibial nerve, lateral sural cutaneous nerve, common peroneal nerve

15. peroneus longus, peroneus brevis; superficial peroneal

IV. Answer questions briefly

1. The cervical plexus is formed by the anterior branches of the first 4 cervical nerves (C_{1-4}). The brachial plexus is formed by the anterior branches of the lower 4 cervical (C_{5-8}) and great part of the 1st thoracic nerve (T_1). The lumbar plexus is formed by the anterior branches of the first 3 lumbar nerves, a part of the last thoracic nerve and the 4th lumbar nerve. The sacral plexus is formed by the lumbosacral trunk, which is composed of 5th and a part of the 4th lumbar nerve, the anterior branches of the sacral and coccygeal nerves.

2. The anterior branch contains mixed fibers and supplies the structure of the limbs and the lateral and ventral parts of the trunk. The posterior branch contains mixed fibers and supplies the muscles and skin of the posterior parts of the neck, thorax, back, sacral region and gluteal region. The meningeal branch is a small branch, runs backward the vertebral canal to supply the dura mater. The communicating branches are connected with the sympathetic trunk.

3. The lesser occipital nerve is distributed to the skin behind the auricle and the occipital region. The great auricular nerve is distributed to the skin around the auricle and much of the external ear. The transverse nerve of neck is distributed to the skin of the anterior part of neck. The supraclavicular nerve has 3 branches which are distributed to the skin at the upper portion of the chest, the base of the neck and the shoulder.

4. The musculocutaneous nerve innervates the anterior group of muscles, which are biceps brachii, brachialis and coracobrachialis. The radial nerve innervates the posterior group of muscle, which is triceps brachii.

5. The femoral nerve innervates the anterior group of muscles, which are sartorius and quadriceps femoris. Pectineus, one of the medial muscles is also innervated by the femoral nerve. The obturator nerve innervates the medial group of muscles, which are adductor longus, adductor brevis, adductor magnus and gracilis. The sciatic nerve innervates the posterior group of muscles that are biceps femoris, semimembranosus and semitendinosus.

6. The symptoms of the injury of axillary nerve include: paralysis of muscles of deltoid

and teres minor; numbness over the lateral side of the upper part of the arm. The explanation of the symptoms is that the muscular branch of the axillary nerve innervates the deltoid and teres minor and its cutaneous branches control the sensation of the skin of the lateral side of the upper part of the arm.

7. Injury of the femoral nerve results in paralysis of muscles of quadriceps femoris displaying impaired flexion of the hip joint and a loss of sensation on the skin of the anterior aspect of the thigh and the medial side of the leg and foot. The explanation of the symptoms is that the muscular branch of the femoral nerve innervates the quadriceps femoris and sartorius and its cutaneous branches control the sensation of the skin of the anterior aspect of the thigh and the medial side of the leg and foot.

8. The deep peroneal nerve innervates the anterior group of muscles, which are tibialis anterior, extensor halluces longus and extensor digitorum longus. The superficial peroneal nerve innervates the lateral group of muscles, which are peroneal longus and peroneal brevis. The tibial nerve innervates the posterior group of muscles, which are gastrocnemius, soleus, tibialis posterior, flexor halluces longus and extensor digitorum longus.

V   Answer questions in detail

1. On each side, there are 12 thoracic nerves. The upper 11 lie in intercostal spaces and are called the intercostal nerves, and the 12th lies below the last rib and is called the subcostal nerve. Muscle branches of these nerves supply the intercostales and anterolateral abdominal muscles. The cutaneous branches are distributed to the skin of the thoracic and abdominal wall. The distribution of the anterior branches of the 12 pairs of thoracic nerves is segmental. On the anterior surface of the trunk, they present about the levels as follows:

T_2— the sternal angle, T_4— the nipple, T_6— the xiphoid process, T_8— the costal arch, T_{10}— the umbilicus, T_{12}— the anterior superior iliac spine.

2. The sciatic nerve is the largest nerve in the body and is divided into tibial nerve and common peroneal nerve in the popliteal fossa. Before bifurcation, the sciatic nerve gives off the muscular branches, supplying the posterior compartment of the thigh, including biceps femoris, semimembranosus and semitendinosus.

The muscular branches of the tibial nerve innervate the posterior group of muscles that are gastrocnemius, soleus, tibialis posterior, flexor halluces longus and flexor digitorum longus. The cutaneous branch of the tibial nerve, the medial sural cutaneous nerve, joins the sural nerve that is distributed to the skin of the posterior and lateral surface of the leg and over the lateral border of the dorsum of the foot.

The common peroneal nerve is divided into thesuperficial and deep peroneal nerves at the level of the neck of the fibula, besides the lateral sural cutaneous nerve. The muscular branches of the superficial peroneal nerve innervate the lateral group of muscles, which are peroneus longus and peroneus brevis. The cutaneous branch of superficial peroneal nerve is distributed to the skin of the distal part of the anterior lateral surface of the leg, the dorsum of the foot and toes. The muscular branches of the deep peroneal nerve innervate the anterior group of muscles, which tibialis anterior, extensor halluces longus and extensor digitorum longus. The cutaneous branch of deep peroneal nerve is distributed to the skin between the first and second toes.

Chapter 24   The Cranial Nerves

Ⅰ. **Single choice**

1. A	2. D	3. A	4. D	5. C	6. B	7. C	8. B	9. B	10. A
11. B	12. A	13. D	14. B	15. A	16. B	17. A	18. B	19. C	20. B
21. A	22. A	23. C	24. B	25. D	26. B	27. A	28. D	29. A	30. D
31. B	32. D	33. C	34. C	35. B	36. B	37. D	38. A	39. C	40. B

Ⅱ. **Double Choices**

1. AE	2. BC	3. CD	4. AC	5. AB	6. BE	7. CD	8. AD	9. BD
10. AC	11. CD	12. AB	13. AC	14. BC	15. BE			

Ⅲ. **Fill the blanks**

1. ganglionic, optic canal, middle
2. oculomotor nerve, trochlear nerve, abducent nerve, ophthalmic nerve
3. glossopharyngeal nerve, vagus nerve, accessory nerve
4. ciliary, ciliary muscles, sphincter pupillae
5. the general somatic sensory, the special visceral motor, ophthalmic nerve, maxillary nerve, mandibular nerve
6. pterygopalatine ganglion, submandibular ganglion, lacrimal, submandibular, sublingual
7. temporal branch, zygomatic branch, buccal branch, marginal mandibular branch cervical branch
8. the special somatic sensory, vestibular ganglion, cochlear ganglion
9. jugular foramen, otic ganglion, parotid
10. the general somatic sensory, the general visceral sensory, the general visceral motor, the special visceral motor
11. hepatic branch, anterior gastric branch, posterior gastric branch, celiac branch
12. trochlear, abducent, oculomotor
13. chorda tympani, lingual
14. the special visceral motor, jugular foreman, trapezius, sternocleidomastoid
15. the general somatic motor, hypoglossal canal

Ⅳ. **Answer questions briefly**

1. The oculomotor nerve innervates the levator palpebrae superioris, the superior rectus, the inferior rectus, the medial rectus and inferior obliquus. The trochlear nerve innervates the superior obliquus. The abducent nerve supplies the lateral rectus.

2. In abdomen, the left vagus nerve becomes anterior vagal trunk which is divided into hepatic branches and anterior gastric branches two major terminal branches. The right vagus nerve becomes to posterior vagal trunk that is divided into posterior gastric branches, celiac branches two major terminal branches.

3. The ganglion related to the oculomotor nerve is ciliary ganglion. The ganglia related to the facial nerve are the pterygopalatine ganglion and submandibular ganglion. The ganglion related to the glossopharyngeal nerve is the otic ganglion. The ganglia related to the vagus nerve are intramural ganglia and paramural ganglia.

4. The trochlear nerve contains the general somatic motor fibers and supplies the superior obliquus. The abducent nerve contains the general somatic motor fibers and supplies the lateral rectus. The accessory nerve contains the special visceral motor fibers and supplies the sternocleidomastoid and trapezius. The hypoglossal nerve contains the general somatic motor fibers and supplies all the intrinsic muscles and extrinsic muscles of tongue.

5. The sensation of tongue includes the taste sense controlled by the chorda tympani nerve of the facial nerve (anterior 2/3 of tongue) and the lingual branch of the glossopharyngeal nerve (posterior 1/3 of tongue); general sense controlled by the lingual nerve of the trigeminal nerve (anterior 2/3 of tongue) and the lingual branch of the glossopharyngeal nerve (posterior 1/3 of tongue).

   The movement of tongue is controlled by the hypoglossal nerve.

6. The temporal branches supply the occipitofrontalis and orbicularis oculi. The zygomatic branches supply the orbicularis oculi and the zygomaticus. The buccal branches supply the buccinators, orbicularis oris. The marginal mandibular branch supplies the muscles of the lower lip. The cervical branch supplies the platysma.

7. The special visceral sense includes the taste and smell. The taste is conveyed by the chorda tympani nerve of the facial nerve (anterior 2/3 of tongue) and the lingual branch of the glossopharyngeal nerve (posterior 1/3 of tongue). The smell is conveyed by the olfactory nerve.

8. The masticatory muscles include the temporalis, the masseter, the medial and lateral pterygoid muscles, and they are supplied by the mandibular nerve of the trigeminal nerve.

   The muscles of pharynx and larynx are stylopharyngeus, cricothyroid, transverse arytenoid, the oblique arytenoid, the thyroarytenoid and posterior cricoarytenoid, which are supplied by the glossopharyngeal nerve and vagus nerve.

Ⅴ. **Answer questions in detail**

1. There are 7 fibrous components in the cranial nerves as below: the general somatic sensory fibers, the general somatic motor fibers, the special somatic sensory fibers, the general visceral sensory fibers, the general visceral motor fibers, the special visceral sensory fibers and the special visceral motor fibers. The 12 pairs of cranial

nerves are classified into 3 groups:

The sensory nerves include olfactory nerve, the optic nerve and the vestibulocochlear nerve.

The motor nerves include the oculomotor nerve, the trochlear nerve, the abducent nerve, the accessory nerve and the hypoglossal nerve.

The mixed nerves include the trigeminal nerve, the facial nerve, the glossopharyngeal nerve and the vagus nerve.

2. The ciliary ganglion is related to the oculomotor nerve, and its postganglionic fibers supply the sphincter pupillae and ciliary muscles. The pterygopalatine ganglion is related to the facial nerve, and its postganglionic fibers supply the lacrimal gland and the glands of the nose and palate. The submandibular ganglion is related to the facial nerve, and its postganglionic fibers supply the submandibular and sublingual glands. The otic ganglion is related to the glossopharyngeal nerve, and its postganglionic fibers supply the parotid glands. The intramural ganglia and paramural ganglia are related to the vagus nerve, and its postganglionic fibers supply the smooth muscles, cardiac muscles and glands of the viscera in the thoracic and abdominal cavities.

3. The CN I (olfactory nerve) passes through cribriform foramina in cranial cavity. The CN II (optic nerve) passes through optic canal in cranial cavity. The CN III (oculomotor nerve), IV (trochlear nerve), the ophthalmic nerve of the CN V and CN VI (abducent nerve) pass through the superior orbital fissure in/out of cranial cavity. The axillary nerve of the CN V (trigeminal nerve) passes through foramen rotundum in cranial cavity and the mandibular nerve of the CN V passes through foramen ovale in/out of cranial cavity. The CN VII (facial nerve) passes through facial canal and stylomastoid foramen in/out of cranial cavity. The CN VIII (vestibulocochlear nerve) passes through internal acoustic meatus in cranial cavity. The CN IX (glossopharyngeal nerve), X (vagus nerve) and XI (accessory nerve) pass through jugular foramen in/out of cranial cavity. The CN XII (hypoglossal nerve) passes through hypoglossal canal out of cranial cavity.

Chapter 25   The Visceral Nervous System

I. **Single choice**

    1. D   2. A   3. C   4. C   5. B   6. C   7. A   8. D   9. A   10. D

    11. B   12. D   13. D   14. A   15. D   16. C   17. D   18. B   19. D   20. C

II. **Double Choices**

    1. CD   2. CD   3. AB   4. BD   5. AC   6. BD   7. CD   8. AD

III. **Fill the blanks**

    1. sympathetic nerve, parasympathetic nerve

    2. $T_1 - L_3$ segments of spinal cord

    3. paravertebral ganglia, prevertebral ganglia

4. paravertebral ganglia, interganglionic branches

5. brainstem, sacral spinal cord

6. ciliary ganglion, pterygopalatine ganglion, submandibular ganglion, otic ganglion

7. E-W nucleus, superior salivary nucleus, inferior salivary nucleus, dorsal nucleus of vagus nerve

8. white communicating branches, gray communicating branches

Ⅳ. **Answer questions briefly**

1. The lower center of sympathetic nerve is located in the lateral horn of spinal cord at $T_1 - L_3$, and there are paravertebral and prevertebral ganglia. There are 19 to 24 pairs of paravertebral ganglia, celiac ganglion, superior mesenteric ganglia, inferior mesenteric ganglia aorticorenal ganglia, etc.

2. The lower center of parasympathetic nerve is located in the brainstem and the sacral parasympathetic nuclei of S_{2-4}. The parasympathetic nuclei in the brainstem include the oculomotor accessory nucleus, the superior salivary nucleus, the inferior salivary nucleus and the dorsal nucleus of vagus nerve. The parasympathetic ganglia include paraorganic and intraorganic ganglia. The paraorganic ganglia include ciliary ganglion, submandibular ganglion, pterygopalatine ganglion and otic ganglion.

3. The sympathetic preganglionic fibers refer to fibers originate from the lower center of sympathetic nerve and relay in the corresponding ganglia. There are three directions for sympathetic preganglionic fibers entering the sympathetic trunk: ① terminates at the corresponding paravertebral ganglia; ② rises or falls within the sympathetic trunk, and then terminates at the upper or lower paravertebral ganglia; ③crosses the paravertebral ganglia to terminate and relay within the prevertebral ganglia.

4. The parasympathetic nuclei in the brainstem include the oculomotor accessory nucleus, the superior salivary nucleus, the inferior salivary nucleus and the dorsal nucleus of vagus nerve.

5. The greater splanchnic nerve consists of preganglionic fibers passing through the 5th to 9th thoracic paravertebral ganglia, passing through the crus of diaphragm and terminating in the celiac ganglion. The lesser splanchnic nerves consist of preganglionic fibers passing through the 9th to 12th thoracic sympathetic ganglia, passing through the diaphragmatic foot and terminating at the aorticorenal ganglion.

Ⅴ. **Answer questions in detail**

1. The lower center of sympathetic nerve is located in the lateral horn of spinal cord at $T_1 - L_3$, and there are paravertebral and prevertebral ganglia. There are 19 to 24 pairs of paravertebral ganglia, and the prevertebral ganglia include celiac ganglion, superior mesenteric ganglia, inferior mesenteric ganglia aorticorenal ganglia, etc.

The lower center of parasympathetic nerve is located in the brainstem and the sacral parasympathetic nuclei of S_{2-4}. The parasympathetic nuclei in the brainstem include the oculomotor accessory nucleus, the superior salivary nucleus, the inferior salivary nucleus and the dorsal nucleus of vagus nerve. The parasympathetic ganglia include paraorganic and intraorganic ganglia. The paraorganic ganglia include ciliary ganglion, submandibular ganglion, pterygopalatine ganglion and otic ganglion.

2. Lacrimal gland: The preganglionic fibers come from the superior salivary nucleus and transfer to the pterygopalatine ganglion via the greater petrosal nerve of the facial nerve.

　　Submandibular and sublingual glands: Preganglionic fibers originate from the superior salivary nucleus and reach the submandibular ganglion through the chorda tympani of the facial nerve.

　　Parotid gland: The preganglionic fibers come from the inferior salivary nucleus and transfer to the otic ganglion via the lesser petrosal nerve of the glossopharyngeal nerve.

Part 6　The Endocrine Organs

Ⅰ. **Single choice**

　　1. D　　2. A　　3. C　　4. B　　5. C　　6. C　　7. B　　8. D　　9. A　　10. A

　　11. A　　12. D　　13. B　　14. C　　15. B

Ⅱ. **Double Choices**

　　1. BE　　2. CE　　3. DE　　4. AE　　5. AE

Ⅲ. **Fill the blanks**

　　1. endocrine organs, endocrine tissues

　　2. hormone

　　3. hypophysis, pineal body

　　4. adenohypophysis, neurohypophysis

　　5. hypothalamus

　　6. thyroid gland, parathyroid gland

　　7. lateral lobes, isthmus, pyramidal lobe

　　8. thymus

　　9. semilunar shape, triangular shape

　　10. islets

Ⅳ. **Answer questions briefly**

　　1. A secretory gland without excretory duct is called endocrine gland. The substance secreted by such gland is called hormone, which directly enters the blood circulation and acts on its target. Endocrine glands include pituitary gland, pineal body, thyroid gland, parathyroid gland, suprarenal gland, etc.

　　2. The pituitary gland is located in the pituitary fossa of the sphenoid bone. It can be di-

vided into two parts: adenohypophysis and neurohypophysis. Among them, the former includes the distal part, the intermediate part and the tuberous part; the latter includes the nervous part and the infundibulum. The adenohypophysis secretes the somatotropin, gonadotropin, thyrotropin, adrenocorticotropin, follicles stimulating hormone and luteinizing hormone, etc. The neurohypophysis only stores vasopressin and oxytocin.

3. The thyroid gland is located in the neck, in front of the larynx. It is butterfly-shaped or "H"-shaped with two lateral lobes and isthmus between them. The isthmus is located in front of 2 – 4 tracheal cartilage rings. The upper end of the lateral lobe can reach the middle part of the lamina of thyroid cartilage. In some people, there is a pyramidal lobe above the isthmus.

4. The adrenal glands is located on superior medially of both kidneys and are enclosed by renal fascia. The left adrenal gland is semilunar shape and the right one is triangular. The arteries of the adrenal gland includes: the superior suprarenal artery, which originates from the inferior phrenic artery; the middle suprarenal artery, which originates from the abdominal aorta; and the inferior suprarenal artery, which originates from the renal artery.

V. Answer questions in detail

(1) The endocrine system includes a group of endocrine tissue and organs.

(2) The endocrine organs have no ducts — "ductless glands", the secretions are conveyed by the blood circulation.

(3) Each endocrine gland can secrete one or more types of hormones acting on the target cells or organs.

(4) They have a rich supply of blood vessels.

(5) The quantity of each hormone is less, but has a specific and wide effect.

References

[1]FANG XIUBIN,HU HAITAO. A Textbook of Human Anatomy[M]. Changchun:Jilin
   Science and Technology Press,2008.
[2]ROBERT CAROLA,JOHN P. HARLEY, CHARLES R. NOBACK. Human Anatomy
   and Physiology[M]. New York:McGraw-Hill Publishing Company,1990.

References